I0790294

TABLE OF CONTENTS

INTRODUCTION

Chinese cuisine encompasses a variety of culinary traditions that originated in China. Thanks to the Chinese diaspora and the country's historical influence, Chinese cuisine has had a significant impact on various other Asian and international cuisines, often adapting to suit local tastes. Today, staple ingredients of Chinese cuisine, such as rice, soy sauce, noodles, tea, chili oil, and tofu, as well as essential utensils like chopsticks and woks, can be found worldwide. In this book, you'll learn step by step guidelines on how to prepare sumptuous Chinese food!

ESSENTIAL COOKING UTENSILS

The delectable flavors of Chinese cuisine have long been influenced by the expertise of chefs and the tools they employ in their cooking. By utilizing these cooking utensils, you can prepare a multitude of your beloved Chinese dishes in the comfort of your own home. Some of them include:

1 A wok
2 A cutting board
3 A Chinese Scoop Strainer
4 A wok shovel
5 Steaming baskets
6 Cleaver
7 A ladle
8 Long and ordinary chopsticks
9 Rice Cooker
10 Pressure Cooker

ESSENTIAL CHINESE INGREDIENTS

The culinary practice of Chinese cuisine is often regarded as an artistic endeavor, and its deep-rooted legacy can be fully appreciated through the prevalent use of traditional Chinese ingredients in contemporary cooking. Some of them include;

1 Dark soy sauce
2 Shaoxing Wine
3 Cornstarch
4 Soy sauce (Regular or White)
5 Scallions
6 Oyster sauce
7 Sesame oil
8 White pepper (grounded)
9 Garlic
10 Ginger

DISCLAIMER

Please note that it is the reader's responsibility to carefully review the listed ingredients before cooking, ensuring that none of them may cause potential adverse effects for those consuming the food. Adverse effects may include allergies, health-related restrictions, and pregnancy-related effects. The nutrition information provided for the recipes in this book is an estimate and should be used for guidance purposes only.

CHAPTER 1

NOODLES

There are numerous ways to prepare Chinese noodles, and they complement meats and vegetables exceptionally well. These noodles are simple to make and can be quickly transformed into delicious dinner-time meals.

Chinese noodles exhibit a wide range of variations based on the region of production, ingredients used, shape or width, and method of preparation. Originating in China, noodles hold a vital role as an essential ingredient and staple in Chinese cuisine. They form a significant part of regional cuisines across China and are also embraced in countries with substantial overseas Chinese communities. Chinese noodles can be crafted from wheat, buckwheat, rice, millet, oats, beans, potatoes, sweet potatoes, and even fish. Today, there are more than 1,200 commonly consumed types of noodles in China, with countless additional noodle dishes incorporating these varieties.

Moreover, Chinese noodles have made their way into the culinary traditions of neighboring East Asian countries like Korea and Japan, as well as Southeast Asian nations including Malaysia, Singapore, Indonesia, Vietnam, Cambodia, the Philippines, and Thailand.

TYPES OF NOODLES
1.1. Lamian Noodles
1.2. Dao Xiao Mian Noodles
1.3. Saang Mein Noodles
1.4. Lai Fun Noodles
1.5. Yi Mein Noodles

1.1 LAMIAN NOODLES
This is quite common in China and other parts of Asian countries. A good number of people cook it. It can also be deep-fried with meat and vegetables.

To prepare Lamian, beaches are created by stretching and folding the dough, performing in fibrous and leathery polls. The dough consists of water, salt and wheat flour.

 Most frequently, people cook it to make a succulent coliseum of instant noodles. They also deep- fry it with meat and vegetables.

To make Lamian, the chef creates beaches by stretching and folding the dough, performing in fibrous and leathery polls. The dough is made of wheat flour, swab, and water.

The more the dough us folded, the thinner the noodles can get. The method was introduced by Song Xu (1504).

Making Lamian can be relative from one place to the other . In Lanzhou, more pressure is put on the noodles. But in Beijing, it is done in a gentler way.
Lamian polls can be used for other dishes. A good example is Tangmian which is a beef soup. People use it to make chow mein, a veritably notorious pate dish. People use Lamian to make salads with tattered cucumbers and tomatoes.

Lamian also has artistic significance. There are Hui ethnic families in Northwestern China who retain the Lamian caffs in China, and they only make Halal food, which doesn't contain pork.

There's also another variety of Lamian called " Shandong Lamian, " which belongs to the Shandong fiefdom.

INGREDIENTS FOR LAMIAN NOODLES
1 2 cups (280 g) of Bread Flour or All Purpose Flour
2 ¼ cup of Oil
3 1 tsp of Salt
4 2/3 cups (160 g) of Warm Water

STEP BY STEP INSTRUCTIONS

1 Dough Preparation: If kneading by hand, mix flour and salt in a bowl. Gradually add water and mix until there is no loose flour visible. Briefly knead the mixture into a dough, cover it, and let it rest for 10-15 minutes. Knead again for approximately 2 minutes until the dough becomes very smooth.
If using a stand mixer, add flour, salt, and water to the mixing bowl. Knead on low speed until a smooth dough forms.

2 Coating and Resting the Dough: Divide the dough into two parts; let them be equal. Then, flatten each piece into a rectangle shape, about ½ cm thick. You can use a rolling pin to flatten. Coat each piece with oil, place them one by one on a tray, and then cover with cling film. Allow the dough to rest for 1.5 hours.

3 Cutting the Dough: Bring a large pot of water to boiling point. While you are waiting for the water to boil, you can cut your dough. Place one piece of dough on a chopping board and cut it widthways into strips. For round, thin noodles, cut them to be approximately 1 cm wide. For flat, wide noodles, cut them to be about 3 cm wide.

4 Pulling the Noodles: Gently pick up one strip of dough by holding each end. Pull it towards opposite directions in a smooth and consistent motion.
While your arms move apart, bounce the noodle against the worktop to help it stretch. further. Fold the noodle and repeat this pulling motion.

5 Cooking the Noodles: Drop the pulled noodle into the boiling water. Repeat the procedure for other strips cut from the first piece of dough.
Cook the thin noodles for about 1 minute, or the wide noodles for approximately 2 minutes. Meanwhile, cut the second piece of dough into strips.
Using a pair of chopsticks, transfer the cooked noodles to a serving bowl.

6 Repeating for the Second Batch: Repeat the process of pulling and cooking for the second piece of dough.

7 Serving the Noodles: To prevent the noodles from sticking together, serve them immediately.

8 Storage: If not served right away, rinse the noodles briefly with cold water and add a few drops of sesame oil. Stir well and store in the refrigerator for up to 2 days.

9 Reheating: When ready to reheat, bring a pot of water to a boil. Add the noodles and cook for no more than 30 seconds.
Please note that you can add broth or mix the noodles with toppings and dressings according to your preference.

1.2 DAO XIAO MIAN NOODLES

This bean means " knife- cut noodles ". It's a delicacy of Shanxi terrain. The way people prepare it is amazing. The culinarians shave cornucopia of wide strands of pates from a large dough. They put the strands in a pot of boiling water. especially, their hands move truly snappily. They always use sharp cutters to ensure that the process runs fluently. The strands are not always steady, but they taste perfectly tough. The culinarians have excellent timing chops. They have to let each beachfront stay in the pot until it's ready to eat. And do you know that Dao Xiao Mian Noodles are one of the most ideal bean types for making ramen? Yes, they are.

INGREDIENTS FOR DAO XIAO MIAN NOODLES

For the Dough:
1;3 cups of all purpose flour
2 1 cup rice flour
3 1 teaspoon baking powder
4 2 cups of water
5 1 teaspoon salt

For the Soup:
6 1 1/2 lb ground meat
7 1 cup dried shrimp soaked for an 1 hour or more
8 10 cup water
9 6 teaspoons minced garlic
10 3 tablespoons crab paste

STEP BY STEP PROCEDURE

1 Mix everything together and knead into a dough. Knead it for 10- 15 minutes. If it's too soft, add a little more flour. It should not be too soft though.

2 Let it rest for another 15 minutes. papule water to shave noodles in. Stay and do the haze first.

3 Mix the ground meat with 2 tablespoons of oyster sauce, 2 ladles fish sauce,1/2 tablespoon navigator,1/2 tablespoon sugar, 2 tablespoon oil painting oil oil painting,1/2 tsp ground pepper, and 2 ladles of the diced garlic.

4 Mix this well so the meat sticks together. In a pot, heat 2 tbsp of oil. Add in the 2 tsp diced garlic and stir to help burn. When turning brown, add in the dried shrimps.

5 Don't dispose off the water in order to use it after you stir the shrimp a little. Now add in the water. Let the haze bring to boil and also turn the fire down to let it poach.

6 In another visage/pan, heat about 2 tbsp of oil and add in the grouser paste. Stir it and also add in the meat. Stir until it's partial chef and also add into the haze.

7 Bring the haze to a boil and also add in the taste.

1.3 SAANG MEIN NOODLES

Another type of thin noodles is Saang Mein noodles. People make the beaches with tapioca flour, potassium carbonate, wheat flour, swab, and water. Thanks to the thin beaches, it gets tender veritably snappily. It's smooth and has an adulatory texture and wheat flavour.

People frequently serve it on its own or add sesame oil or vegetables to it. A veritably common type of vegetable used is kai- lan.
Saang Mein noodles are more popular in Hong Kong culinary culture than in mainland China. You can also find it in Chinatowns in other countries.

INGREDIENTS

1 Wheat flour
2 Water
3 Tapioca flour
4 Salt
5 Potassium carbonate

A MORE ELABORATE LIST OF INGREDIENTS

1 2 fresh wonton noodles, loosen
2 2- 3 tbsp cuisine oil for cooking
3 3 cloves garlic
4 1/2 carrot, hulled and julienned
5 1 cabbage splint, julienned
6 3 Chinese or shitake mushrooms,   rehydrated and thinly sliced
7 2 fishcake, thinly sliced
8 1 spring onion, cut into 1 inch length
9 A sprinkle beansprouts, irrigated and drained
10 8 king prawns, hulled and deveined with tails complete
11 1/2 tsp gusto wine
12 1/2 tbsp dark soy sauce
13 1 tbsp light soy sauce
14 1/2 tsp funk stock grains(not compulsory)

STEP BY STEP PROCEDURE

1 Marinate prawns with the gusto wine

2 Bring a large pot of water to the pustule. Once boiling, add the noodles and cook for 10- 15 seconds. After that, wash the noodles in cold water. Drain well.

3 In a wok, toast the oil over medium high heat. Add the garlic and cook for about 2-3 minutes, until smoothly golden. Add the mushrooms and stir for about 1 minute.
Also add the carrot and cabbage and cook for a farther minute. Add the fishcake and prawns and cook for about 30 seconds, after which you place the noodles, stirring constantly. Season with dark soy sauce, light soy sauce and funk stock grains and cook for about 1- 2 minutes, until the noodle is cooked through.

4 Eventually, add the spring onions and beansprouts and give it a quick stir, about 30 seconds, until cooked.

5 Serve instantly with some pickled green chillies. Garnish with some heated white sesame seeds.

Take note that If you can not get fresh egg noodles, you can substitute for dried thin egg noodles. You can also add funk, pork, roasted duck or smoked duck strips.

1.4 LAI FUN NOODLES

It is also known as Thick Rice Noodles. In Malaysia, they are referred to as Laksa Noodles.
Lai Fun noodles originate from the Pearl River Delta region of China. Outside China, you can also find it in Chinatowns.
The noodles are made from rice flour and tapioca bounce. They come in short and long forms. They're slightly leathery. Numerous people confuse Lai Fun noodles and silver needle noodles. They're both thick and white. You can distinguish them by paying attention to the ends. The ends of Lai Fun noodles aren't phased like silver needle's.
A good number of people use this type of noodles to prepare soups and stir- fried dishes.Making Lai Fun noodles is a pleasurable process.

INGREDIENTS

1 1 Cup (120 grams) Rice Flour
2 1 Cup of Boiling Water
3 1/2 tsp Sea Salt
4 2 Tbsp Potato Starch
5 1 Tbsp Vegetable Oil

STEP BY STEP PROCEDURE

1 Dry Shindig rice flour over low heat for about 15-20 minutes or until smooth and light.

2 Then, transfer it into a mixing bowl and gradually add in the hot water.

3 Mix in the potato brio, mix well and then gather the dough with a rustic spoon.

4 When it's slightly cool but still warm, knead the dough until smooth and elastic, about 8 to 10 minutes.

5 Prepare a bowl or cold surge or ice water, and set down.

6 Bring a pot of water to a boiling point and add some sea-salt.

7 Put a piece of dough into a potato platform or murukku maker, press to push out the noodle onto the boiling water.

8 Cook the rice noodles for about 2 minutes, or until they rise up.

9 Gently remove the noodles with a line strainer, and transfer to the ice/ cold water. Repeat with the remaining dough. Drain the rice noodles and give them a thorough rinse under cold running water. The rice noodles should be used the same day or stored in the fridge for about two days.

1.5 YI MEIN NOODLES

It can also be called Longevity noodles.. They've a pivotal part in Chinese occasions like birthdays, lunar new time dinners, and marriages. These noodles are thought to bring good luck and substance.
Yi Mein noodles are made of wheat flour, eggs, and sodium bicarbonate or soda pop water. The beaches have a pleasurable unheroic colour and a spongy and leathery texture. After making the beaches, the culinarians deep- fry them, also dry them and shape them into a cutlet.
Put it in mind that this noodle can easily become soggy after being cooked. So make sure that you do not overcook them. The best way to get their perfect texture is to boil them for lower than 3- 4 minutes before you use them to make any dish.
This type of noodle is also veritably protein. You can use it to make your favorite Chinese delectables similar as salads and mists. I love to stir fry it with my favourite meat and veggies.

INGREDIENTS

1 31/4 of water
2 12 ounces of Yimein noodles
3 Salt
4 1 tbsp of hot water
5 8 ounces of Chinese chives that are thinly sliced (Green and white)
6 2 tsp of regular soy sauce
7 2 tbsp of oyster sauce
8 1/2 tsp of sesame oil
9 Freshly ground white pepper
10 3-4 tbsp of vegetable oil
11 5 shiitake mushrooms that are thinly sliced
12 1/8 tsp of sugar
13 2 tsp of dark soy sauce

STEP BY STEP PROCEDURE

1 Begin by cooking the noodles for 3-4 minutes in hot water.

2 Drain them and set them away.

3 Combine the sugar with 1 teaspoon of hot water and whisk until the sugar dissolves.

4 Mix in soy sauce, dark soy sauce, oyster sauce, sesame oil painting, and pepper to combine.

5 Sauté the chives(the green part) for 30 seconds over high heat, including the mushroom.

6 Add and stir the noodles at this point. You can also add more oil if necessary, and cook for 20-30 seconds.

7 Then, stir the noodles and the sauce. Let both cook for like a minute.

8. Pour the remaining chives, and cook for another 2-3 minutes, or as preferred.

CHAPTER 2

DIM SUM

Dim sum can be termed a traditional delicacy of small plates served in teahouses. So, like tapas(for the Spanish), you get all kinds of dishes to partake with musketeers and family.
And it happily begins with the tea!
You 'll order a pot for the table, then choose from a variety of inconceivable dim sum fashions, like delicious cakes, wontons and fumed dumplings.
Let's get into some of this sumptuous recipes!

2.1 Chinese Steamed Chicken Buns
2.2 Air Fryer Dumplings
2.3 Steamed BBQ Pork Buns (also called Car Siu Bao)
2.4 Sichuan Spicy Wonton in Red Oil
2.5 Fried Shrimp Balls

2.1 CHINESE STEAMED CHICKEN BUNS

Buns that are fluffy and pillowy, filled with tasteful funk and vegetable filling! Sounds super delicious, doesn't it? Yeah right!
These are just as sumptuous like char siu buns, but the funk filling makes them a healthier option – just 179 calories per serving!
The technical part of making stuffed fumed buns is the folding aspect. You need to ensure that you have just enough stuffing so each of them look dainty and inviting.

INGREDIENTS

1 140 g each- purpose flour
2 50 g wheat starch
3 1 tablespoon cold water
4 4 g active dry incentive or instant incentive
5 80 ml lukewarm water
6 1 teaspoon of oil
7 1 tablespoon baking powder
8 45 g pulverized sugar

Fillings for the chicken

1 225 g skinless and boneless chicken breast (chopped into smaller sizes)
2 1 teaspoon diced scallion
3 1/2 mug finely sliced napa cabbage
4 1/4 tablespoon of salt
5 1/4 tablespoon of chicken bouillon powder
6 1 tablespoon fish sauce
7 1/2 tablespoon sugar

8 3 dashes white pepper
9 1 tablespoon cornstarch
10 2 dried shiitake mushrooms(soak in hot water to soften, also minced into thin strips)

STEP BY STEP PROCEDURE

1 Sift the flour, the powdered sugar and the wheat starch. Then, transfer the content to a mixing bowl. Make a well at the centre of the flour mixture then, add the warm water and salt. Dissolve the yeast with water, then gently bring the flour mixture together and add in the oil.

2 Knead the dough with your hands for about 10- 15minutes or until the dough is soft. It should look smooth after this.

3 Then, cover the dough and let it rise for an hour or until it increases in size. Ensure you cover the dough with a damp cloth.

4 Using cold water, dissolve the baking powder. Then, sprinkle over the dough and knead until they are well combined. Roll up the dough into a cylinder shape. After this, divide the dough into 8 equal parts.

5 Next, mix all the ingredients of the chicken filling together. After this, put it aside.

6. Using a rolling pin, try to flatten each dough to a 3" circle. Place a portion of the chicken filling right in the middle.

7 Wrap the dough and fold it up.

8. Then, enclose the opening by pinching and twisting the dough. Ensure the top of the chicken bun is sealed tight.
Place it then on a 2" x 3" piece of paper(parchment paper). Repeat the process until you make like 8 buns.

9. After, then arrange the chicken buns on your steamer. While doing this, leave about 1 gap in between the various buns. Steam on high heat or in a preheated steamer for 8-10 minutes. You can add a tablespoon of Chinese white ginger, if you prefer, to give the chicken buns a white colour.

10 After, remove the buns from the steamer, serve instantly.

Note that you can add some drops of white ginger into the hot water to make the chicken buns whiter. Another ingredient that can make the chicken buns whiter is like juice. You can add some drops.

2.2 AIR FRYER DUMPLINGS

You 're in for a nice treat! These Air Fryer Dumplings gather together quickly without having to thaw them,which is quite easy! If you have not tried air-frying frozen dumplings before, This system is great. It also works for gyoza, wontons, and frozen potstickers. Also, to get crisp dumplings, you don't need to worry about oil splatter.

I love crisp dumplings but I dislike having to deal with oil splatter. Thanks to the air fryer, you can now get crisp dumplings without having to worry about oil splatter. Also, there's no need to flip them to get each side to crisp up. The air fryer makes it easy to make crisp dumplings.
At times, there's just not enough time to cook from the beginning.
When this happens, you can always rely on a bag of frozen dumplings to do the work.
Simply put them in the air fryer and let the air fryer do its work!
In a few minutes, you'll get juicy and sumptuous dumplings.
This equally works on homemade dumplings that you've frozen beforehand.

INGREDIENTS

1 Frozen dumplings
2 Oil spray

STEP BY STEP PROCEDURE

1 First of all, place the frozen dumplings inside the basket(air fryer basket). Then, Spray sufficiently with oil to ensure all the sides are well oiled.

2 Air fry the frozen dumplings for 8 minutes. It should be at 375F. Shake the basket and continuously air fry for 2-3 minutes or to your taste of crispiness.

2.3 STEAMED BBQ PORK BUNS (ALSO CALLED CHAR SIU BAO)

Soft and fluffy Char Siu Bao, also known as Chinese Steamed BBQ Pork Buns, feature a delightful combination of juicy and sweet Chinese BBQ pork (char siu) encased in tender and fluffy steamed buns. These buns can also be baked to perfection, offering a classic pastry option found in Chinese bakeries. The light and airy bun serves as a delectable wrapper for the irresistible filling, which consists of Chinese BBQ pork, shallots, flavorful sauces, and aromatic spices. Prepare to indulge in the mouth-watering blend of sweet and savory flavors that these buns have to offer.

INGREDIENTS

Filling:
1 400 gr Chinese bbq pork about 1 lb, dice into small pieces.
2 1 Tbsp soy sauce
3 1 small onion peeled and finely chopped
4 1 tsp red yeast rice powder optional, for red color
5 1 Tbsp cooking oil
6 1 tsp ginger grated or finely chopped

Seasonings for filling:
1 2 Tbsp all-purpose flour
2 1 Tbsp hoisin sauce

3 1 tsp dark soy sauce (optional)
4 1 Tbsp oyster sauce
5 3 Tbsp sugar
6 1 tsp sesame oil
7 Salt to taste

STEP BY STEP PROCEDURE

Making the stuffing(can be made ahead)

You should mix all the constituents for seasonings in a bowl, except the flour though. After this, put it aside.
Then, preheat your wok over high heat.
After that, add the oil. Also add onions and gusto and saute until they are all soft. It can take about 3-5 minutes. Then, add the BBQ pork(or uncooked chicken meat if you are using that), and cook until the colour changes to opaque). Add the seasonings and red yeast rice powder (that is if you are using it). Then, stir to blend. Sprinkle in the flour.
The pork admixture will start to thicken and glue together. Taste to know if the sugar is enough. If not,add more sugar.
It should be sweet, rather than savoury. Turn the heat off and let it fully cool down before wrapping.

Wrapping

 Once you have the basic dough, divide them into 12 equal pieces. Sprinkle flour on your work surface. Work with one dough at a time and let the remaining one be covered. Use your plan to flatten the dough, then, with a rolling pin, create a circle of about 4-6 inches. Let the middle part be slightly thicker. The reason is to support the weight of the filling. Also, let not the dough be too thin. This is because of the dough is too thin, the steamed buns might wrinkle later when you steam.

For round shape

Put about 1-2 tbsp of housekeeper siu filling at the centre and gather the edge together to enclose into a round ball. Then, place the seam side down. Use both of your palms to cup the dough and move the dough in a circular form to give it a taller shape. This part is very important so that instead of your steam buns spreading to the sides after storming, they come out tall.

Place it on a piece of parchment paper. Then, with some milk, smoothly dab the face of the bun and use your cutlet to smoothen the face. Then cover with a clean cloth to help drying. So the same for the other doughs.

IF YOU WISH TO PLEAT SOME PATTERNS

Place the char siu filling at the centre. Then, make a fold around the edge and also pinch to seal. Use both of your palms to cup the dough and move the dough in a circular form to give it a taller shape. This part is very important so that instead of your steam buns spreading to the sides after storming, they come out tall.

Then, place on a piece of parchment paper. If you have patterns, there's no need to dab the surface with milk. Gently cover with a saran wrapper to hinder drying. Do the same with another dough.

Proofing

Allow the shaped buns to proof until it doubles the original size (or 50% double).. They actually don't necessarily have to double in size. This may occur in about 15 minutes. Just observe to make sure the buns have puffed up to ½ of its original size and that it feels lighter, before steaming, else the buns will be kind of tough. Also, do not overproof them.

Steaming

Most probably your steamer might not be suitable to accommodate steaming all the buns at once. You may need to get it done in like 2- 3 batches. This means, while waiting for the steamer, the rest of the batches will likely sit longer and continue to proof. This is not a good one for the buns! What then should be done? Ensure to cover them with plastic wrap and immediately place them in the refrigerator to stop the yeast activity, or reduce it at the least instance, until ready to be steamed.

Let the water in the steamer boil to the highest point. Then, wrap the cover with a cloth, in order to prevent water trickling from the lid,and in turn, creating burn spots. Place some of the buns on the steamer. Reduce the heat to medium. Close the lid, but not completely in order to let some steam escape. Steam for about 15 minutes on medium heat. Then, turn off the heat and wait for 5 minutes before removing the steamed to a cooling rack. This will help the bottom from getting wet and even soggy.

Storing

So, if you have plans to store them, once the steam is off the buns, place them on a baking sheet and let them not touch each other. Then, put them inside the freezer for like 60 minutes before transferring them to a freezer bag.

Reheating

They can likewise be reheated in the steamer without thawing. You can steam over high heat for about 5 minutes.

2.4 SICHUAN SPICY WONTON IN RED OIL

This sumptuous recipe yields the most tasty hot sauce, just like the road food you would get in Sichuan.
If you 're looking for red oil wontons like the type you will find in a small hole- in- the- wall restaurant in Sichuan, then here it is. This form is different from various spicy wonton recipes you might have seen. This method also guarantees maximum satisfaction with that real- deal Sichuan flavor.

The sauce consists of chili oil,ginger, onions, soy sauce and gusto. So it's not just pure heat but a wonderful combination of flavors as well.

INGREDIENTS

1 60 small wonton wrappers , thawed (or if you prefer, 40 large wonton wrappers)
2 Aromatic water
3 1/4 teaspoon salt
4 1 teaspoon Sichuan peppercorns
5 2 green onions , sliced
6 1 tablespoon ginger , minced
7 1/4 cup boiling water

Sauce

1 1 1/2 tablespoons Chinkiang vinegar
2 1/4 cup flavored sweet soy sauce (or more if you prefer a sweeter dish)
3 2 teaspoons garlic , grated
4 2 green onions , sliced
5 1/2 cup homemade chili oil plus 4 teaspoons chili flakes from the oil

Filling

1 2 teaspoons cornstarch
2 1/2 lbs (225 g) pork , minced
3 1/8 teaspoon white pepper powder
4 1 large egg

Garnish

1 A few tablespoons of boiling water from cooking the wontons (This is optional)
2 Chopped cilantro, toasted ground Sichuan peppercorn flakes, plus toasted sesame seeds for garnish (This is also not compulsory)

STEP BY STEP PROCEDURE

1 Firstly, prepare the aromatic water. Put all the ingredients for the aromatic water in a little bowl. Stir it well and let it infuse for about 15-20 minutes. Strain all the solid ingredients. You can discard them later.

2 Prepare the sauce (red oil sauce). Put all the ingredients for the sauce in a bowl. Then, Stir it well.

3 Make the wontons. Add the diced pork in a bowl. Then, include the aromatic water, white pepper powder, cornstarch and egg. Mix it very well until a smooth and sticky paste is formed.

4 Work on the wontons one after the other. Then, place about ½ or 1 tablespoon filling(1 tablespoon filling is for bigger wontons) on the third of the wrapper(the lower third). After this, try to fold the bottom side over the stuffing. Also, roll the filling to the other side of the wrapper. Ensure to put a little layer of egg white on the end of the wonton wrapper. Then, bind the two ends and press them together in order to lock in the filling in the wrapper. After this, Place in a plate, and let the width be like a finger apart.

5 When you have done about 10-15 wontons, ensure that cover them with a damp paper towel in order to help them from drying out.

6 Know that you can store your wonton for a day in the fridge, or even freeze them for a month! Yes it's possible. If you want them freeze them, seal with plastic wrap, the tray of wontons and place in the freezer. When the wontons become solidly frozen, you can then transfer them from the freezer to an airtight bag. It works!

7 Cook and assemble. Put a good amount of water in a pot to boil. Then, add the wontons, like 15-20 at once. Stir gently to prevent them from sticking down.You can stir with a spatula. Cook well until the wontons are floating on top. It should take like 3-5 minutes. Then,begin to transfer the wantons into each bowl; like 6-8 wantons at a time. Pour the hot broth and sauce(about 2 tablespoons each) and then serve.

8 Coat the wontons with sauce by mixing them very well.

Store

Know that you can store your wonton for a day in the fridge, or even freeze them up for a month! Yes it's possible. If you want them freeze them, seal with plastic wrap, the tray of wontons and place in the freezer. When the wontons become solidly frozen, you can then transfer them from the freezer to an airtight bag. It works well

To cook frozen wonton

Boil a good amount of water on high heat. Then, add the wontons. Stir, albeit, gently to help from sticking. Cook until the water reaches a boiling point again. Gently turn the heat to medium. After this, cover your pot but not completely, to prevent it from overboiling. Keep boiling for about 2-3 minutes (3 minutes is for larger wontons). Closely monitor the broth, and if you see that it starts to boil over, quickly uncover and stir. After this, replace the cover. Keep cooking for like a minute or two or until the wontons are completely cooked.

2.5 FRIED SHRIMP BALLS

These are delicious and juicy shrimp balls that are covered by tiny cubes of bread which are fried perfectly. These dim sum crisp fried shrimp balls are quite easy to make and are really enjoyed by both kiddies and grown-ups. It's a very good way to use up stale bread. You can air fry or deep fry your shrimp balls; it all depends on you.

This sumptuous dim sum delicacy is made up of a mixture of shrimp with seasonings and aromatics which are shaped into balls, and then coated with bread (cut into cubes). You can also coat it with strips of spring roll sheet; either way, both work.

INGREDIENTS

For shrimp balls:
1 250 gr peeled and deveined shrimp
2 ½ tsp sesame oil
3 1 tsp fish sauce
4 1 tsp cornstarch
5 ⅛ tsp ground white pepper
6 ½ tsp chicken powder
7 ¼ tsp salt
8 ¼ tsp sugar
9 1 stalk green onion
10 Oil for frying

Coat with:
1 180 gr bread slices or more as needed, cut into small cubes

STEP BY STEP PROCEDURE
1 Preparing the shrimp balls. To prepare the shrimp balls, you'll need about 340- 350 grams of unpeeled shrimp. Peel and the shrimp and remove the veins. Place it in a food processor and then pulse for some time in order to give it a paste consistency. Then, mix the other ingredients together, cover it and allow it to marinate for like an hour or even overnight.

2 Assembling. **Coat** the shrimp balls with white sandwich bread. You can also use any bread of your choice though. When it is ready to be assembled, trim off the crust from the bread and cut it into like 1/ 2- 1 inch cubes.

3 Take about 2-3 tablespoons of the shrimp mixture (you can take more than that if you want a bigger size) and mold it into a ball. Your palms should be slightly wet in order to prevent sticking. Then, roll it on the bread cubes and ensure that the surface is fully covered by the bread cubes. Squeeze a bit with your palms to ensure that the bread cubes are well attached to the sticky shrimp mixture, in order to prevent them from falling off while cooking.

Air-fried version

To air-fry, you have to brush the bread cubes with little oil and arrange them gently into the air-fryer basket. Then, air-fry for like 5 minutes at 350 F (180C). Rotate it so that they can brown evenly. Continue to air-fry for the next 2-4 minutes. The colour in the outside should change to golden-brown and it should be well cooked inside also.

Deep-fried version

To do this, preheat a little oil to fry. The oil should cover half of the shrimp balls at least while frying. To know if the oil is ready, pit a skewer into the oil; and if bubbles gather around it, then the oil is ready. Begin to put the shrimp balls into the oil and move then around so they won't burn and will fry evenly. Keep frying for about 2-3 minutes or until it changes colour to golden-brown. After it changes colour, remove to a paper towel and keep on frying the rest.

CHAPTER 3

CHINESE SAUCES

Chinese cooking offers a delightful array of flavors, thanks to the abundant use of rich condiments in its dishes. Whether it's soy sauce or rice wine, these essential sauces are indispensable for an authentic culinary experience that you won't want to miss out on.

3.1 Hot Chili Oil
3.2 Sweet and Sour Sauce
3.3 Hoisin Sauce
3.4 Soy Sauce
4.5 Plum Sauce
3.6 Hot Mustard

3.1 HOT CHILLI OIL

Chili oil is a mixture of oil that is spice-infused and crunchy, plus hot chili flakes! Aside from its hotness, another important feature is in its distinguished fragrance and aroma.

INGREDIENTS

1 2-3 tbsp gochugaru Korean Chili Powder
2 1/2 tbsp sesame seeds
3 1-2 tsp Szechuan pepper (i grounded mine using a mortar and pestle), add more or less if you want more of the numbing spice
4 1/2 tsp Chinese five spice powder
5 1/2 tsp fine salt
6 1 cup neutral oil (avocado, vegetable, canola, etc)
7 1 tsp sugar
8 2 tbsp chili flakes or crushed red pepper

STEP BY STEP PROCEDURE

1 Add all ingredients in a bowl (exclude the oil though). Then, mix them well.

2 In the meantime, place the neutral oil in a saucepan and heat over medium heat. Keep that up until small bubbles start to appear and the oil gets hot; that should be around 250F/ 120C. You can test how hot the oil has gotten by dropping some chili flakes to see if it sizzles. If it does, then the oil is hot enough. You can also test the hotness of the oil by dipping a chopstick (wooden

one) and it should gather bubbles. However, the oil is hot enough If it does. Completely turn off the heat and also instantly add oil to the chili mix.

3 Mix gently and thoroughly. Then, have a taste of the sediments and you can season with more sugar and/or salt to taste, if you so require. You can add in more chili powder if you are a fan of spice.

Storage

Allow the mixture to cool down before you transfer it to a jar(ensure the jar has a lid). Seal the jar tight and store it in a cool, dry place with room temperature. Each time you want to take some of the chili oil, use a clean spoon in order to prevent any form of contamination. It can be kept for about 3-6 months. It largely depends on how fast and soon you consume the chili oil.

3.2 SWEET AND SOUR SAUCE

This sumptuous sauce is quick, easy and a perfect condiment for your own very fried chicken!
It is made up of a fruity base with rice vinegar that provides the sour, and also brown sugar adding in the sweet. It gets thick with a cornstarch slurry which brings the whole thing to the thick, gelatinous consistency which is a major requirement in my mind.
It is easy and quick to make. It is great on standard fried chicken which can create one of the best plates of sweet and sour chicken you'll eat. It can also accompany some of your favorite DIY Chinese-takeout dishes.

INGREDIENTS

1 1 tablespoon cornstarch (about 1/4 ounce; 7g)
2 1 tablespoon (15ml) soy sauce
3 2/3 cup (160ml) pineapple juice
4 1/3 cup (74g) light brown sugar
5 3 tablespoons (45ml) ketchup
6 1 tablespoon (15ml) water
7 1/3 cup (80ml) rice vinegar

STEP BY STEP PROCEDURE

1 Mix in a bowl, water and cornstarch. Then, set it aside.

2 In a saucepan (like a medium-sized one), add soy sauce, rice vinegar, ketchup and brown sugar and let them boil over medium heat. Stir and cook until it is thick. This should take about 1-3 minutes.
You can now remove it from heat and use it immediately.

STORAGE

If you don't want to use all immediately, you can store it up in the refrigerator (in an airtight container) for about 2 weeks at most.

3.3 HOISIN SAUCE

This home made sauce has so much sumptuous flavours because it is sweet and rich! It's so rich that you might reconsider buying from a store again!

INGREDIENTS

1 1/4 cup soy sauce
2 1 teaspoon cornstarch
3 2 teaspoons sesame oil
4 1 tablespoon rice vinegar
5 2 garlic cloves finely minced
6 2 teaspoons sriracha sauce
7 1/4 teaspoon ground pepper
8 1 Tablespoon water
9 3 Tablespoons molasses
10 2 Tablespoons peanut butter

STEP BY STEP PROCEDURE

1 Mix together, in a saucepan, sesame oil rice, soy sauce, pepper, molasses, vinegar, garlic, peanut butter and sriracha.

2 Mix water and cornstarch together in a little bowl. Then, transfer it into the sauce. Let it simmer until it thickens. Then, remove it from the heat and allow to cool down.

3.4 SOY SAUCE

This sweet sauce originates from China and has been used in Asia for so long a time. Soy sauce can go with different cuisines.

INGREDIENTS

1 16 ounces organic high-quality soy beans
2 16 tablespoons salt
3 24 tablespoons or 12 ounces of multipurpose flour
4 1 gallon fresh water

STEP BY STEP PROCEDURE

There are three important steps you need to take note of here;
1 Making the Koji
2 Fermenting the brine, and
3 Refining the final product.

1 Pour about 3-4 cups of water into a pot to cook the soy beans if they are not yet cooked. Then, add beans and bring all to a boiling point. After the water boils, reduce the heat a little and allow it to simmer. Keep cooking for about 1 hour or 1 ½ hours or until soft and tender and until they

are partially removed from their pods. For faster cooking, you can make use of a pressure cooker too.

2 After it has cooked, put the soy beans in a food processor and let it blend to a paste. Pour the pureed beans into a bowl and combine it with flour.

3 Place and put the bean-flour mixture on a clean surface and shape it into a log. Then, cut the log into some slices. It can be about ¼-inch in thickness.

4 Then, arrange the sliced soy bean on a damp paper towel and cover them with another wet paper towel. Cover well in cling wrap and then put it away in an unobtrusive area in your kitchen. Allow it to sit there for about 7 days or until you notice that the discs are covered in mold.

5 After the above, remove the wrap from the discs and arrange them on a baking sheet to prevent them from touching one another. Leave each of them to get dried in direct sunlight. Their colour should change to brown when dry. This, then is the koji.

6 Now, let's discuss fermentation. For this, take a pot that you might not be needing soon. Pour in salt and water and stir to combine. Then, add the soybean discs and cover. The purpose of this step is to allow the discs to dissolve in the salt water. This can actually take up to 6 months. Ensure to stir the mixture daily.

7 When all the soybean slices have dissolved completely, strain the mixture into bottles for storage. You can use cheesecloth to strain. After this, the soy sauce is ready to be used. You can use the soy sauce to flavor your meats, soups, veggies and even seafood.

3.5 PLUM SAUCE

Indulge your taste buds with the smooth, sweet, and tangy Chinese plum sauce that captivates with its intricate blend of traditional Chinese spices. This delectable sauce offers a mesmerizing flavor profile, leaving you wanting more! Its versatility shines through as it can be used as a dip, stir-fry sauce, basting sauce, or glaze. You can even toss it with noodles or drizzle it over rice for an effortlessly delicious meal. Plums hold a significant role in Chinese culture, with the Chinese being credited as the first cultivators of this beloved fruit.

INGREDIENTS

1 2 pounds plums, pitted and chopped
2 1 star anise
3 1/2 cup brown sugar, lightly packed
4 3 tablespoons freshly grated ginger
5 2 garlic cloves
6 1/2 cup cider vinegar
7 1/4 cup soy sauce

STEP BY STEP PROCEDURE

1 Prepare. Combine the soy sauce, vinegar, ginger, brown sugar, garlic, and star anise in a large pot, and bring to a boiling point. Reduce the heat a little and let it simmer until it is thick. It should

take like 20-25 minutes. Fish out the star anise and then discard. Then, purée the sauce with a stick blender.

2 Refrigerate. Scoop it into jars or into bowls. You can cover and refrigerate for like 3 weeks.

3 Adopt the boiling-water method. Scoop into clean, half-pint canning jars, leaving about 1/4 inch of headspace. Then, release the trapped air. After that, wipe clean the rims; the centre lids on the jars and then screw on jar bands. Process it for about 10 minutes. Turn off the heat and remove the canner lid. After that, let the jars rest in the water for about 5 minutes. Remove the jars and set them aside for about 24 hours. Then, check the seals. After, store in a cool, dark place. You can store it for about 6-12 months.

3.6 HOT MUSTARD

Hot Mustard is by far the easiest, yet mist fascinating sauce ever!

INGREDIENTS

1 3 tablespoons hot mustard powder, such as Colman's
2 3 tablespoons cold water

STEP BY STEP PROCEDURE

1 Mix together water and mustard powder in a bowl until they are completely combined. Then,let it rest for about 15 minutes. After this you can use it immediately.

CHAPTER 4

TOFU AND VEGETABLES STIR FRY

Over the past few years, there has been an increase in the availability and popularity of certain tofu products in the Western market, including deep-fried tofu and savory tofu. These ready-to-eat options have gained traction due to their milder taste, making them more appealing to Western consumers. Compared to traditional plain tofu, which is less familiar to Westerners in terms of preparation and texture, these tofu variations have been met with greater acceptance.

Textural Attributes

One of the advantages of tofu is its versatile texture, allowing it to be sliced into small pieces and molded into various forms for different dishes. The textural properties of tofu play a crucial role in assessing its overall quality and acceptability. For instance, firm tofu tends to be harder and more cohesive, requiring more effort to break down its structure. On the other hand, tofu with high springiness often exhibits higher elasticity and increased chewiness, making it more challenging to consume.

Therefore, the factors influencing the development of tofu's three-dimensional network structure are closely linked to its textural characteristics.

As previously mentioned, the composition of glycinin (11S) and β-conglycinin (7S), their content ratio (11S/7S), and their subunit profiles directly influence the formation of tofu's network structure and, consequently, its textural attributes.

INGREDIENTS

1 454 grams of medium-firm tofu, recommended for a soft texture
2 3 cups of broccoli, cut into florets
3 1 ½ cups of carrots, peeled and diagonally sliced
4 1 ½ cups of snap peas, ends sliced off
5 ½ tablespoon of minced garlic
6 1 ½ cups of water
7 ¾ cup of vegetable oil

Stir-Fry Sauce:

1 3 tablespoons of oyster sauce (or substitute with vegetarian stir-fry sauce for vegan or vegetarian options)
2 2 tablespoons of regular soy sauce (not light or dark)
3 1 teaspoon of sesame oil
4 1 teaspoon of Shaoxing Cooking Wine (optional, can be omitted to avoid alcohol)
5 1 cup of water
6 2 tablespoons of cornstarch

STEP BY STEP INSTRUCTIONS

1 Begin by slicing the block of tofu in half vertically. Then, slice both strips into 1 cm thick squares. For a thicker tofu with a softer interior, slice into 2 cm thick squares. Place the tofu squares on a paper towel-lined plate to absorb excess liquid, and then transfer them to a smooth plate without a lip.

2 In a small bowl, whisk together the ingredients for the stir-fry sauce.

3 Heat a wok or non-stick pan over high heat (275 degrees F) with cooking oil. To check if the oil is hot enough, insert a wooden chopstick and look for bubbles. Once bubbles appear, it's time to fry. Carefully lower the plate with the tofu into the pan using a spatula, being cautious of oil splatter. Fry the tofu on both sides until golden crispy brown, approximately 5 minutes. Keep an eye on the bottom of the tofu to determine when to flip it. Use a slotted spoon to transfer the fried tofu to a paper towel-lined plate to absorb excess oil. Set aside.

4 Remove most of the cooking oil from the pan, leaving approximately 1 teaspoon. Heat the pan over medium-high heat and add minced garlic, carrots, broccoli, and snap peas. Stir-fry the vegetables for a few minutes. Pour in the water and let it simmer until the greens become vibrant and tender.

5 Once the vegetables have softened, gently mix in the fried tofu, allowing it to sink to the bottom and absorb the liquid, becoming soft again. Cook for an additional 5 minutes until the tofu is soft.

6 Reduce the heat to medium. Whisk the stir-fry sauce in the bowl again to incorporate any cornstarch that may have settled at the bottom, and pour it over the vegetables and tofu. Gently mix everything together until well incorporated

7 Increase the heat to high and continue cooking, stirring regularly, until the sauce thickens and is no longer runny, for approximately 8-9 minutes. Monitor the sauce for the desired thickness. Transfer the dish to a serving plate and enjoy it while hot!

CHAPTER 5

CHINESE DESSERTS

Chinese cuisine is renowned for its delectable rice and noodle dishes, bursting with savoury and umami flavours. Yet, the realm of Chinese desserts is equally captivating, if not more so, than its savoury counterparts.

Discover an array of mouthwatering Chinese desserts that can elevate your meal experience. By introducing these delightful treats, you can add depth and variety to your menu, avoiding the monotony of repetitive desserts.

CHINESE COOKIES
1 Delight in the crunch of Almond Cookies.
2 Enjoy the nutty goodness of Chinese Sesame Cookies.
3 Indulge in the buttery Chinese Walnut Cookies.
4 Unfold a surprise with Fortune Cookies

CHINESE DESSERTS WITH PUDDINGS
5 Indulge in the lusciousness of Mango Pudding.
6 Savour the delicate Tau Foo Faa (Soybean Pudding).
7 Delight in the richness of Eight-treasure Rice Pudding.
8 Experience the comforting flavours of Chinese Steamed Egg Puddings

CHINESE CAKES
9 Enjoy the delightful Red Bean Cake
10 Try the delicate and flaky Snowflake Cake.
11 Discover the unique taste of Mung Bean Cake.
12 Celebrate with the traditional Chinese New Year Cake.
13 Indulge in the festive Mooncake.
14 Treat yourself to the soft and creamy Chinese Steamed Custard Buns (Nao Wong Bao).

CHINESE TARTS
15 Experience the smoothness of Egg Tarts.
16 Savour the tangy sweetness of Pineapple Tarts.
Fried Chinese Desserts:
17 Delight in the unique texture of Fried Milk.
18 Enjoy the crispy perfection of Fried Bananas.
19 Satisfy your cravings with Sachima.
20 Bite into the crispy exterior of Sesame Seed Balls.

CHINESE DESSERT SOUPS
21 Warm up with the soothing Chinese Sweet Potato Ginger Soup.
22 Relish the sweetness of Dessert Soup Red Bean Soup.

OTHER AMAZING CHINESE DESSERTS
23 Relish the unique taste of Pineapple Buns.
24 Explore the fluffy and aromatic Fa Gao.
25 Quench your thirst with the refreshing Bubble Tea.
26 Celebrate with the chewy Glutinous Rice Balls (Tang Yuan).

Some of these amazing desserts will be discussed here! Let's go!

5.1 ALMOND COOKIES

Discover the secrets to crafting delectable Chinese almond cookies boasting a delightful buttery essence and a delicate, satisfying crunch. Surprisingly, this recipe is easier than you may anticipate! Indulge in a batch to commemorate the lunar new year or savour them alongside a soothing cup of tea.

The distinctive blend of sweetness and nuttiness originates from a trio of almond ingredients. Moreover, the process of creaming butter and sugar creates a heavenly lightness, complemented by a crisp texture which crumbles with each bite. During Chinese New Year, I take immense pleasure in preparing a generous quantity to share with my loved ones, as these festive treats are believed to bring good luck. Furthermore, they keep well for future enjoyment!

INGREDIENTS

1 1 1/3 cups of almond flour (lightly packed)
2 1 cup (2 sticks) of unsalted butter (chilled and cubed)
3 Pinch of kosher salt
4 1 cup plus 2 tablespoons of sugar
5 1 teaspoon of almond extract
6 1 ¾ cups of flour(all-purpose flour)
7 ½ teaspoon of baking soda
8 2 large eggs (separated)
9 Thinly sliced almonds for decoration

STEP BY STEP PROCEDURE

1 Begin by beating the almond flour, salt, and butter. Utilise an electric mixer with a paddle attachment, setting it to medium speed for approximately 3 minutes. The mixture will adopt a coarse and chunky appearance.

2 Break one of the eggs and the almond extract, gently mixing them on low speed until they are just combined.

3 Proceed by sifting the flour, sugar, and baking soda, adding them to the mixture. Mix slowly until the ingredients are just combined.

4 Refrigerate the dough. Flatten the dough into a disc shape, then wrap it in plastic wrap. Allow it to chill in the refrigerator for two hours.

5 Heat the family oven beforehand and get the baking sheet prepared. Set the oven to 325°F and line a baking sheet with parchment paper.

6 Beat the remaining egg. Take a small bowl and beat the remaining egg until well mixed.

7 Shape the dough into flattened balls on the cookie sheet. Take portions of the dough and roll them into approximately 3/4-inch wide balls. Arrange them on the sheet, leaving about an inch of space between each. Gently press them down with your palm to create a coin shape.

8 Position the slivered almonds and brush the cookies with the beaten egg. Place one slivered almond in the center of each cookie. Next, using either a pastry brush or your finger, brush the surface of each cookie with the beaten egg. This will give the cookies a glossy appearance once they are baked.

9 Bake at 325°F for 13 to 15 minutes, or until the edges begin to develop a light tan colour. Allow the cookies to cool on the baking sheet placed on a wire rack.

5.2. CHINESE SESAME COOKIES

Sesame cookies, similar to almond cookies and other varieties of Chinese cookies, traditionally contained lard. However, this recipe offers a healthier alternative by using a combination of butter and shortening, resulting in cookies with just over 75 calories. To enhance the flavor, consider adding a few tablespoons of toasted sesame seeds to the cookie dough before baking.

INGREDIENTS

1 2 cups all-purpose flour
2 ¼ cup brown sugar
3 ½ teaspoon baking soda
4 ½ cup (4 ounces) unsalted butter, softened
5 ½ cup shortening
6 ¾ cup granulated sugar
7 ¼ teaspoon salt
8 1 teaspoon almond extract
9 1/3 to ½ cup white sesame seeds (as desired)
10 ¾ teaspoon baking powder
11 1 large egg

STEP BY STEP PROCEDURE

1 Start up by gathering together the necessary ingredients.

2 In a medium bowl, sift together the flour, baking soda, salt and baking powder.

3 In a large bowl, use an electric mixer to cream together the softened butter, shortening, and both white and brown sugars.

4 Add the egg and almond extract to the mixture, and continue beating until well combined.

5 Gradually add the flour mixture into the bowl, ensuring thorough mixing. The dough may appear dry and crumbly at this stage.

6 Use your fingers to shape the mixture into a cohesive dough. Then, form the dough into two rolls or logs, each approximately 10 to 12 inches in length.
Wrap them tightly and refrigerate for at least 2 hours, preferably 4 hours. (Alternatively, you can prepare the dough ahead of time and refrigerate it overnight).
By following these steps, you'll be able to enjoy these delicious sesame cookies that offer a healthier twist on the traditional recipe.

7 Ensure to preheat your oven to 325°F.

8 Take one of the dough logs and gently score it at ¾-inch intervals, creating 15 pieces. Cut along the scored lines.

9 Shape each piece into a small ball and roll it in a bowl of sesame seeds, ensuring the ball is fully coated. (Note: If desired, you can brush the ball with lightly beaten egg before dipping it in the sesame seeds to help them adhere to the cookie).

10 Place the sesame seed-coated balls onto a lightly greased cookie tray, ensuring there is approximately 2 inches of space between each ball.

11 Bake the cookies in the preheated oven at 325°F for approximately 15 to 17 minutes. They are ready when a fork inserted in the center comes out clean and they can be easily lifted from the baking sheet. Allow the cookies to cool down completely.

12 Once the cookies have thoroughly cooled, you can either enjoy them immediately or store them in a sealed container for later consumption.

5.3. CHINESE WALNUT COOKIES

Chinese walnut cookies, known as hup toh soh, possess a delightful texture that is dry, crispy, and crunchy. These type of cookies offer a subtle sweetness that enhances their overall appeal. They make a fantastic gift for foreign guests and are a cherished snack during the Chinese New Year.

INGREDIENTS

1 2 cups cake flour (270 g)
2 1/4 teaspoon baking powder (2 g)
3 1/2 teaspoon baking soda (3 g)
4 8 tablespoons butter or lard (4 oz or 115g, at room temperature)
5 1/2 cup sugar (115 g)
6 1 egg (beaten and divided; the egg I used weighed about 62 g with shell on)
7 1/2 teaspoon baking soda (3 g)
8 3/4 cup finely chopped toasted walnuts, plus 12 raw walnut halves (75 g)

STEP BY STEP PROCEDURE

1 Start by sifting the cake flour, baking soda, and baking powder together. Set aside the sifted mixture. In a large mixing bowl, cream the butter, sugar, and salt until well combined. Add the finely chopped walnuts to the butter mixture, followed by the majority of the beaten egg (reserve 2 teaspoons for later). Mix them all until a dough forms. It's normal for the dough to be slightly crumbly, but it will come together when worked into a ball.

2 Prepare a baking sheet by lining it with parchment paper. Now, gently divide the dough into 12 parts and roll each part into a ball-like shape. Place the balls of dough on the baking sheet, leaving a couple of inches of space between them. Make sure all the cookies fit on a single pan.

3 Gently press a walnut half into the top of each cookie. Allow the cookies to rest for 15 to 20 minutes, covering them with a clean kitchen towel

4 Meanwhile, heat the oven beforehand to 350 degrees F or 175 degrees C. Once the dough has finished resting, brush each cookie with the reserved beaten egg. You can then bake the cookies for about 20 minutes.

5 Afterward, turn off the oven and let the cookies remain inside for an additional 5 minutes. Gently being out the cookies from the oven and let them cool down. Now they're ready to be enjoyed!

5.4. FORTUNE COOKIES

Making something like this was incredibly enjoyable and effortless, not to mention how delightful they turned out! A useful suggestion is to act swiftly once they're out of the oven, despite the intense heat, as it greatly enhances the final result.

INGREDIENTS

1 1 cup all purpose flour (5 oz by weight)
2 3 large egg whites
3 1/4 tsp almond extract
4 3/4 cup sugar
5 1/4 tsp vanilla extract
6 3 tbsp water
7 1/2 cup butter melted

STEP BY STEP PROCEDURE

1 Preheat your oven to 375 degrees F (190 degrees C). Prepare a sheet pan by lining it with parchment paper or a silicone mat. Also, make sure you have your fortune strips ready.

2 Using a stand mixer or a large bowl with a hand mixer, beat the egg whites and sugar on high speed for approximately 2 minutes until they become frothy. Mix in the melted butter, vanilla extract, almond extract, and water until well combined. Gradually add the flour and mix until it is just incorporated into the batter.

3 Take a tablespoon measure and drop spoonfuls of the batter onto the prepared parchment paper, spreading each portion into a 3-inch circle. It is advisable to work with 2-3 circles at a time as they set quickly, making it challenging to fold more than that.

4 Bake the fortune cookies for approximately 7-8 minutes, or until the edges have a slight browning. It's important to avoid over-browning, as this can cause the cookies to snap when shaping. On the other hand, if they don't brown at all, they may tear instead of snapping.

5 Once a batch of fortune cookies is done baking, take them out of the oven promptly. Immediately flip each circle over and fold it in half, creating a semicircle shape. This is the moment to insert your fortune note into the cookie. Be quick with this step as the cookie will still be hot, and you don't want the paper to stick. Place the semicircle onto the edge of a cup and swiftly fold the ends downwards, crimping them to form the classic fortune cookie shape.

6 To help the cookies cool and maintain their shape, place each one in a muffin tin.

7 Repeat the process with the remaining batter and enjoy your homemade fortune cookies!

5.5. MANGO PUDDING

Indulge in the decadent and velvety mango pudding, brimming with the exquisite taste of fresh mangoes. Its simplicity makes it a perfect dessert for entertaining guests. With just 10 minutes and 5 ingredients, you can create this delightful treat.

INGREDIENTS

1 1 packet (1 tbsp) unflavored gelatin (or agar-agar)
2 1 cup (250ml) coconut milk, evaporated milk, half and half (10% M.F.), or table cream (18% M.F.)
3 Sliced mangoes and shredded coconut to garnish (this is optional).
4 1/2 cup (100g) granulated sugar
pinch of salt
5 1/2 cup (125ml) boiled hot water
6 1 cup (250ml) mango puree

STEP BY STEP PROCEDURE

1 In a medium bowl, vigorously whisk together the gelatin and hot boiled water until all lumps disappear.

2 Add in the sugar and salt and whisk together until fully dissolved.

3 Then, include your cream/coconut milk, and the mango puree, until the mixture gives a smooth texture.

4 Afterwards, turn the mixture into about 3-4 little bowls. Cover them up and put in the fridge for about 2 hours or more before serving.

5.6. TAU FOO FAA (SOYBEAN PUDDING)

Tau Foo Fah, also known as douhua in Mandarin, is a delectable Chinese dessert featuring incredibly soft tofu accompanied by a delicate sweet syrup infused with either ginger or pandan. Alternatively, a brown syrup is sometimes used instead of the clear one. Traditionally enjoyed warm, it is equally delightful when chilled. While Tau Foo Fah was once sold by street vendors, nowadays it is commonly found as part of the dim sum selection in Chinese restaurants.

INGREDIENTS

1 4 cups soy milk (960ml) I used cold store bought unsweetened soy milk
2 ½ cup water (120ml)
3 2 tsp vanilla extract
4 1 tbsp agar-agar powder (6.5g)

SYRUP
1 ¾ cup water (180ml)
2 1 inch ginger (smashed)
3 ½ cup sugar (110g)

STEP BY STEP PROCEDURE

1 In a medium-sized pot, heat soy milk over medium heat. Be vigilant as soy milk can easily burn, resulting in an undesirable burnt taste in your tau foo fah. It may also boil over.

2 In a separate pot, bring ½ cup (120ml) of water to a boil. Add agar-agar powder and stir until fully dissolved. Pour the warm soy milk and vanilla extract into the agar-agar mixture, stirring to combine.

3 Once the mixture reaches a boil, turn off the heat. Strain the mixture into a large pot with a lid.

4 Cover the pot with the lid, wrapping a clean kitchen towel around it.

5 Allow the mixture to cool slightly, then transfer it to the refrigerator and let it set for approximately 2 hours.

6 Combine all the syrup ingredients in a small saucepan over medium heat. Stir until there is no iota of sugar particles.

7 Turn off the heat and remove the ginger.
To serve, use a flat spatula to gently cut thin slices of tau foo fah into small bowls.

8 Add 2 to 3 tablespoons of syrup.

Enjoy your delicious dessert!

5.7. EIGHT-TREASURE RICE PUDDING

Eight Treasure Rice Pudding, a delightful delicacy comprising sticky rice, dried fruits, nuts, and red bean paste, is an essential treat for Lunar New Year celebrations.

INGREDIENTS

1 200 g glutinous rice (aka sticky rice, sweet rice) - about 1 cup

2 1 tablespoon white sugar - or brown sugar

FILLING
1 3 tablespoon homemade red bean paste or shop-bought version

TOPPINGS
1 1 handful mixed dried fruit and nuts - e.g. jujube (Chinese dates), apricot, cranberry, raisins, walnuts, pumpkin seeds, peanuts, etc.

You also need
1 Honey - for serving (this is not compulsory though)

2 ½ teaspoon coconut oil - or butter, neutral cooking oil.

STEP BY STEP PROCEDURE

1 Soak the rice: Rinse glutinous rice thoroughly and put in a bowl. Cover the rice with water and let it soak overnight. Drain the rice well and mix it with sugar.

2 Prepare the toppings: If needed, remove seeds from dried fruits and slice them.
Soak jujubes (Chinese dates), peanuts, lotus seeds, or almonds overnight to soften. You can use other nuts dried fruits without having to soak them.

3 Coat the bowl with coconut oil. Let it be done evenly. You can also use natural cooking oil or even butter. The essence of the coconut oil is to prevent or reduce sticking.

4 Spread some portion of nuts and mixed dried fruits on the bottom of the bowl.

5 Then, you can put a portion of the rice over the nuts and dried fruits. Formulate the red bean paste into something like a cyclical shape and put it on top of the rice. Afterwards, add in the remaining rice and flatten it with a spoon.

6 Pour in enough water to level with the rice. Be gentle to avoid moving the rice around.

7 Steam the pudding. Place the pudding bowl in a steamer basket or on a steamer rack. Fill a wok or pot with water. Steam over medium heat for approximately 50 minutes. Check the water level halfway through steaming to prevent it from drying out.

8 Serve the pudding: Allow the pudding to cool for about 10 minutes.Gently run a knife or spatula along the edges of the pudding to separate it.
Place a serving plate over the bowl, flip it over, and carefully remove the bowl.

9 The rice pudding can be enjoyed warm or at room temperature. If desired, drizzle some honey over it for a sweeter taste.

10 Storage and reheating. Store the rice pudding in the fridge for up to 3 days or in the freezer for up to 2 months (wrap it tightly with cling film once it cools completely). To reheat, steam the pudding for 10 minutes (defrost it beforehand if frozen).

5.8. RED BEAN CAKE

This recipe for Chinese red bean cake creates a traditional sweet dessert made with sweetened red bean paste, sugar, and glutinous rice flour. It has a gooey texture similar to Japanese mochi cake and is incredibly delicious. In the past, red bean cakes were commonly enjoyed during the Lunar New Year as they symbolized good luck and prosperity. The red color of the cake represents fortune and happiness, while the white color symbolizes purity.

INGREDIENTS

1 1 cup glutinous rice flour
2 1 cup red bean paste
3 cooking oil/spray for pan frying
4 ½ cup of hot water

HOMEMADE RED BEAN PASTE INGREDIENTS

1 1 cup of dried red bean
2 3 tablespoons sugar (you can adjust to your taste)
3 1 cup of water to add into the blender, adjustable depending on your desired texture
4 1 tablespoon butter or coconut oil
5 4 cups of water to boil the red beans

STEP BY STEP PROCEDURE

1 To prepare the Red Bean Cake:
Begin by adding hot water to the glutinous rice flour and mix thoroughly until well combined. Knead the mixture until it forms a smooth consistency. Set it aside.

2 Divide the dough into 6 equal portions and shape them into small, flat circles. Place approximately 1 tablespoon of red bean filling in the center of each dough circle. Fold the dough

around the filling, shaping it into a ball. Using a rolling pin, gently flatten it into a thick pancake shape, about ¼ inch thick.

3 Heat a non-stick pan over medium-low heat and add a small amount of cooking oil. Cook the uncooked red bean cakes in the pan, flipping them to ensure both sides are evenly cooked. It takes about 4 minutes per side, so be cautious of burning. Pan fry until they turn a light golden brown.

4 Transfer the cooked red bean cakes to a plate and serve them warm. Enjoy!

FOR HOMEMADE RED BEAN PASTE

1 Begin by soaking the red beans in water overnight or for at least 3 hours.

2 Then, drain and rinse the soaked red beans before adding them to a pot with clean water for cooking.

3 In a saucepan, combine the red beans and 5 cups of water. Bring it to a boil and then reduce the heat to medium-low. Let it simmer for one hour, allowing the flavors to develop. (If you're using a pressure cooker, refer to the manual for the recommended cooking time.)

4 Using a spatula, mash the cooled-down red beans into a smooth paste. Transfer the mashed red beans, along with sugar and oil, into a food processor or blender. Blend the ingredients until a creamy texture is achieved or until you reach the desired consistency. Take a taste and adjust the amount of sugar if necessary. Continue blending until the mixture transforms into a smooth batter.

5 In a non-stick saucepan, add one tablespoon of butter, and heat the filling mixture until it's firmed up. Turn off the heat and remove from it the stove immediately. Refrigerate cooked red beans for at least 2 hours before making a cake.

5.9. CHINESE SWEET POTATO GINGER SOUP

This Sweet Potato and Ginger Dessert Soup is a delightful and fulfilling treat that combines warm spices with buttery vegetables. It serves as a perfect conclusion to your day. With just four simple ingredients, it offers a healthy alternative to satisfy your sugar cravings in no time. Simply peel, boil, and simmer, and relish it either hot or cold for a truly enjoyable experience!

INSTRUCTIONS

1 1 kg / 2.2 lb sweet potato
2 100 g / 0.22 brown sugar slab (or to taste)
3 1 1/2 L / 6.3 US cup water
4 60 g / 0.1 lb ginger (according to your preference)

STEP BY STEP PROCEDURE

1 Crush the ginger by using the flat side of a meat mallet or a large, flat knife such as a cleaver.

2 Peel the sweet potatoes, then cut them into sizable chunks. You can opt for clean slices or employ the cleaver by wedging it one-third of the way and breaking off the remaining portion. This technique adds texture to each bite.

3 Boil water and add the sweet potatoes and crushed ginger. Allow it to simmer on medium heat for 10 minutes.

4 Introduce the brown sugar slabs into the mixture and continue cooking for an additional 5 minutes or until the ingredients have reached the desired level of tenderness.

5 Savor the soup while it's hot or refrigerate it for a refreshing cold treat!

5.10 PINEAPPLE BUNS

It is also called Bolo Bao. Pineapple buns, a sumptuous pastry found in Hong Kong-style bakeries, are a timeless treat. These buns boast a soft, mildly sweet base, crowned with a golden, crispy, and crumbly crust. The recipe provided utilizes readily available ingredients found in any local grocery store.

INGREDIENTS

TANGZHONG
1 20 grams all-purpose flour (2 tablespoons)
2 75 grams water (1/3 cup)

DOUGH
1 safflower or any neutral oil for greasing bowl
2 18 grams granulated sugar (1 1/2 tablespoons)
3 7 grams active dry yeast (2 1/4 teaspoons)
4 490 grams bread flour , (see note 1)
5 80 grams sweetened condensed milk (4 tablespoons)
6 1 large egg
7 145 grams whole milk (1/2 cup + 2 tablespoons)
8 55 grams butter(4 tablespoons), melted
9 3 grams kosher salt (1 teaspoon)

TOPPING
1 55 grams butter (4 tablespoons), at room temperature
2 Egg yolk
3 1/8 teaspoon turmeric
4 135 grams superfine sugar (2/3 cup)
5 1 teaspoon vanilla extract
6 1 tablespoon whole milk
7 120 grams all-purpose flour

8 1/4 teaspoon baking powder

EGG WASH
1 1 large egg
2 1 tablespoon whole milk

STEP BY STEP PROCEDURE

1 Prepare the Tangzhong:
In a saucepan, whisk together the flour and water until the flour dissolves.

2 Set the saucepan over medium heat and stir the mixture consistently. Within approximately a minute, the flour will begin to thicken. It's important to stay attentive during this step to prevent the Tangzhong from burning. Once the flour transforms into a light paste, remove the saucepan from heat.

3 Transfer the Tangzhong to a bowl and allow it to cool. As it cools, it thickens while cooling.

4 Prepare the Dough for Buns:
Take a large mixing bowl and grease it with oil, setting it aside for later use.

5 Heat the milk in a microwave-safe bowl for approximately 40 to 45 seconds. Add the sugar to the milk. Use a thermometer to check the milk's temperature, aiming for around 110°F to 120°F. A slight variation of a few degrees is acceptable.

6 Introduce the yeast to the milk and stir to ensure the yeast is properly hydrated. Allow the mixture to sit undisturbed for 5 to 8 minutes as you prepare the remaining ingredients. Within this time frame, the milk/yeast mixture will begin to foam up.

7 In a bowl that you can mix with, add egg, bread flour,yeast mixture/foamy milk, salt, melted butter, condensed milk, and tangzhong.

8 Attach the dough hook to the mixer and mix the dough on low speed for 8 minutes. If the dough begins to roll away from the dough hook in a few minutes, just turn off the mixer. Try to readjust the dough right back to the center of the bowl and then position the dough hook just right in the middle of the dough. Fix the mixer on the "stir" setting for about 15 seconds before increasing the speed to low.

9 After like 10 minutes, transfer the dough from the bowl onto a surface where you can work on it and knead it a few times. The dough should not be sticky, so there is no need to flour the surface.

10 Shape the dough into a ball and place it in the greased mixing bowl. Cover the bowl with plastic wrap or a silicone mat. Allow the dough to rise in a warm area for approximately 1 hour to 1 hour 30 minutes until it doubles in size.

11 Prepare the Dough for Topping. Place the butter in the bowl of a stand mixer and attach the flat beater. Cream the butter on medium-low speed until it becomes light and fluffy, which usually

takes 1 to 2 minutes. Gradually add the superfine sugar in two batches. The mixture may appear crumbly at this stage, and that's perfectly fine.

12 Next, add the egg yolk, milk, and vanilla to the mixer. Mix on low speed until the ingredients are just combined.

13 In a small bowl, combine the flour, baking powder, and turmeric. Add half of this flour mixture to the bowl with the wet ingredients, and mix on low speed until well combined. Then, add the remaining flour mixture and mix again. Once all the loose flour has been incorporated, increase the speed to medium-low and continue mixing until the dough starts to come together in large chunks.

14 Get out all the dough from the bowl and then place it on a surface where you can work with it. Gather it into a single large ball and transfer it to another bowl. Cover the bowl with a towel or silicone mat while the buns finish proofing.

15 Shape the buns and prepare the baking sheets. Line about two baking sheets with parchment paper.

16 After the dough has doubled in size, gently punch it down to release any excess air. Transfer the dough on to a surface where you can work on them. Divide the dough into two equal portions, weighing approximately 450 to 456 grams each. Place one portion of dough back into the bowl, cover it, and refrigerate it while you shape the first batch of buns

17 Now, divide the remaining dough into six equal pieces, weighing around 74 to 76 grams each. Take one piece of dough and knead it several times to eliminate any air bubbles. Shape the dough into a ball and place it on the lined baking sheet, with the seam side facing down. Each dough ball should have a diameter of about 2 inches. Repeat this process over and over again with the remaining dough.

18 Place the balls of dough under a towel and allow them to rise in a warm location for 30 to 45 minutes until they expand to 1.5 times their original size (approximately 3 inches in diameter).

19 Heat the oven beforehand to 375°F/190°C. If you prefer a more golden appearance for the pineapple buns, set the oven to 385°F (196°C). Make sure to position an oven rack in the center.

20 Apply the topping and proceed with baking. While the buns are undergoing proofing, divide the topping dough into 12 equal pieces (around 27 to 29 grams each). Mould each piece into a ball-like shape.

21 Obtain a plastic storage bag and remove the zipper closure. Proceed to cut the bag along the edges, resulting in two sizable plastic sheets. These sheets will be used to roll the topping.

22 In a small bowl, combine an egg yolk with 1 tablespoon of milk to create the egg wash. Shake the ingredients together until they are well blended.

23 Once the buns have finished proofing, it's time to begin rolling out the topping.

24 Take a portion of the topping dough and place it in the center of a plastic sheet. Try to flatten the dough with your palm. Next, cover the flattened disc with the other plastic sheet. Roll out the dough until it forms a circle with a width of approximately 3.5 to 3.75 inches.

25 Remove the top plastic sheet, carefully flip the topping onto your hand, and peel off the remaining sheet of plastic.

26 Place the topping over one of the buns, ensuring that it does not fully cover the bun. It's important to avoid the topping touching the bottom of the baking sheet as it can burn. Repeat the process of rolling out the topping and draping it over the remaining buns.

27 Use the egg wash to brush the tops of the buns.

28 Bake the buns for approximately 14 to 16 minutes until the tops turn a lightly golden colour.

29 Once the initial batch of buns is in the oven, proceed to prepare and bake the second batch.

30 Allow the buns to cool on the baking sheet for a few minutes before transferring them to a cooling rack.

31 Indulge in the buns while they are still warm, as that is when they are at their most delicious.

CHAPTER 6

RICE

Rice holds immense significance as a staple food in China, where it is widely cherished and commonly consumed alongside other dishes. Moreover, cooked rice offers a multitude of culinary possibilities. It can be stir-fried, steamed, slow-cooked, or even roasted. Various cooking vessels, including pots, clay pots, coconut shells, and bamboo, can be used to prepare it. Furthermore, rice can be paired with a diverse range of ingredients, such as eggs, sausages, different meats, and an assortment of vegetables.

Let's consider some of the types of rice
1 Cheese Baked Rice
2 Hainanese Chicken Rice
3 Coconut Rice
4 Yangzhou Fried Rice
5 Braised Rice with Spareribs

6.1 CHEESE BAKED RICE

Baked cheese rice is a beloved dish adored by countless individuals. Its roots trace back centuries to a rich history of cultural fusion, where variations of cheese and rice emerged even during the Middle Ages! This delightful culinary creation is both straightforward and scrumptious, featuring a harmonious blend of rice, cheese, vegetarian ham, and vegetables. It can be prepared using leftover rice or by cooking fresh rice and crowning it with cheese before serving. With a handful of basic ingredients, you can swiftly whip up this expedient and delectable recipe in your kitchen.

INGREDIENTS

1 1 nos broccoli (cut into small florets)
2 1/2 cup mozzarella cheese
3 1 nos carrot (sliced thinly)
4 1 onion (chopped)
5 1 clove garlic (minced)
6 mozzarella cheese for baking

7 1 tsp oregano
8 300 ml cooking cream
9 2 1/2 cup of rice
10 1/2 cup milk
11 1/2 cup water
12 1/2 cup Parmesan cheese
13 1 box brown button mushrooms (sliced)
14 salt or seasoning to taste

STEP BY STEP PROCEDURE

1 Begin by cooking the rice either three hours prior to preparing this recipe or overnight.

2 In a heated pan, add oil and start by sautéing half of the garlic and half of the onion. Once they begin to fry, incorporate the broccoli, carrot, and a pinch of salt.

3 Stir-fry the vegetables until they are fully cooked. If needed, add a small amount of water to aid in the cooking process. Continue stir-frying until any excess moisture evaporates and the mixture becomes aromatic. Once cooked, set it aside.

4 Heat another pan with oil, then add the remaining garlic and onion. Next, introduce the mushrooms and a pinch of salt, allowing them to cook until they release their natural juices.

5 Pour in the cooking cream and water, bringing the mixture to a boil.

6 Add the parmesan cheese and oregano. If the sauce appears too watery, incorporate a small amount of mozzarella cheese to thicken it.

7 Season with salt according to your taste preference. If it's slightly salty, that's acceptable as the rice itself is plain. Optionally, you can also add vegetable seasoning if desired.

8 Finally, incorporate the remaining vegetables into the sauce.

9 Preparing the Rice for Baking: Preheat the oven to 180°C and let it heat up for 10 minutes.

10 Take a 9-inch square baking pan and transfer the cooked rice into it. Pour the entire sauce mixture over the rice and add the remaining mozzarella cheese. Give everything a good mix.

11 Sprinkle an additional layer of mozzarella cheese on top of the rice, adding more if you prefer.

12 Place the baking pan in the oven and bake for 30 minutes.

13 If you prefer a crispy cheese topping, bake for an additional 10 minutes.

6.2 HAINANESE CHICKEN RICE

Hainanese Chicken Rice (海南鸡) has its origins in Hainan, China, a tropical island situated at the southernmost part of the country. Over the years, Hainan Island has emerged as a popular tourist destination in China, attracting visitors with its scenic beauty and, not least, its delectable Hainanese chicken rice, which has gained widespread acclaim.

INGREDIENTS

FOR THE CHICKEN

1 1 whole chicken 3.5 lbs, 1.8kg, preferably organic
2 2 stalks green onion cut into 1" sections (both green and white parts)
3 4 inch section of fresh ginger peeled and cut into 1/4" slices
4 4 cloves garlic
5 1 tablespoon Asian sesame oil
6 1/4 cup kosher salt for exfoliating (the salt should be used for cleaning and not consumed)

FOR THE RICE

1 2 cups reserved chicken poaching broth
2 2 cloves garlic finely minced
3 1 shallot minced
4 2 tablespoons cooking oil like canola, vegetable, peanut
5 2 cups long-grain uncooked rice
6 1/2 teaspoon sesame oil
7 1 inch section of ginger finely minced (or grated on microplane grater

FOR THE GINGER GARLIC SAUCE

1 2 tablespoons grated fresh ginger
2 1 teaspoon rice or white vinegar
3 2 cloves garlic finely minced
4 1/2 teaspoon salt
5 4 tablespoons cooking oil canola, vegetable, grapeseed

FOR THE CHILLI SAUCE

1 1 tablespoon lime juice
2 1 inch section of ginger peeled
3 2 teaspoons sugar
4 4 tablespoons sriracha chili sauce
5 4 cloves garlic
6 2 tablespoons reserved chicken poaching broth

STEP BY STEP PROCEDURE

1 Start the process by boiling a large pot of water. While waiting for the water to boil, clean the chicken by gently rubbing it with kosher or coarse salt. Rinse the chicken thoroughly, both inside and outside.

2 Pre-boil the chicken: Once the water reaches a vigorous boil, carefully place the chicken into the pot. Allow the water to return to a hard boil and let any impurities rise to the surface. Boil the chicken for 5 minutes. Afterward, discard all the water, including the impurities.

3 Empty the pot and refill it with fresh water, ensuring that the chicken is covered by approximately 1 inch. Add the garlic, green onion, and ginger to the pot. Place the pot over high heat and bring it to a boil. Once boiling, reduce the heat to low to maintain a simmer. Allow the chicken to cook for approximately 30 minutes longer (adjust the cooking time if using a smaller chicken). To check for doneness, insert a chopstick into the flesh beneath the leg and observe if the juices run clear. Alternatively, use a thermometer and insert it into the thickest part of the thigh, avoiding contact with the bone. The temperature though should read a temperature of 160F. As the chicken rests, it will continue to cook and reach a temperature of 165F.

4 Once the chicken is fully cooked, switch off the heat and carefully take the pot off the burner. Without delay, lift the chicken out of the pot and transfer it into a container filled with ice water. This rapid cooling technique will halt the cooking process, resulting in a tender and succulent meat, while also providing the skin with a delightful firm texture. After cooling, gently dry the chicken using paper towels, and proceed to rub sesame oil all over it. This step will aid in preventing the chicken from becoming dry.

SEASON THE SOUP

Remove the garlic, ginger, and green onion from the soup. Add salt according to your taste preferences, and season the soup accordingly.

COOK THE RICE

1 Take a large bowl and place the rice in it. Fill the bowl with water and use your hands to swish the water around, rinsing the rice. Tilt the bowl to discard the water while keeping the rice in the bowl. Repeat this process three more times until the water appears less cloudy.

2 Heat 2 tablespoons of cooking oil in a wok or pot over medium-high heat. Once hot, add the ginger, shallots, and garlic, and sauté them until a heavenly aroma fills your kitchen. Be careful not to let the aromatics burn. Add the drained rice and stir to coat it with the oil. Cook for an additional minute. Finally, add the sesame oil and mix well.

3 Pour 2 cups of the reserved poaching broth into the pot and bring it to a boil. Once boiling, reduce the heat to low, cover the pot, and let it cook for 15 minutes. Afterward, remove the pot from the heat and allow it to sit, with the lid still on, for an additional 5-10 minutes.

4 While the rice is cooking, prepare the sauces and carve the chicken in readiness for serving.

PREPARE THE SAUCES

1 For the chili sauce: Using a blender, combine the ingredients for the chili sauce and blend until you achieve a smooth and vibrant red consistency.

2 For the ginger garlic sauce: Heat cooking oil in a small saucepan until it becomes very hot and wisps of smoke start to appear. Turn off the heat and promptly add the garlic and ginger. Allow them to sizzle for a few seconds before stirring in salt and vinegar.

6.3. COCONUT RICE

Enhancing the flavor of rice often involves experimenting with various cooking liquids. While water is commonly used, you can opt for different types of stock to infuse flavours like chicken or mushroom into the rice.

Personally, I enjoy pairing coconut rice with Malaysian, Thai, Lao, and other Southeast Asian dishes. This rice has a delicate hint of coconut aroma, offering a subtly sweet taste. To complement it perfectly, toasted coconut flakes are a must-have ingredient, so resist the temptation to exclude them. They add the ideal finishing touch to this delightful side dish.

INGREDIENTS

1 2 cups jasmine rice
2 1 teaspoon salt
3 2 teaspoons sugar
4 ¼ cup toasted coconut flakes
5 13.5 oz. coconut milk

STEP BY STEP PROCEDURE

1 Begin by soaking the rice in water for 15 minutes, then drain it. Take a medium-sized pot and transfer the drained rice into it. Using a wet measuring cup with a capacity of 2-4 cups, pour in the can of coconut milk and add water until the total liquid volume reaches just under 2 cups. Add this mixture to the pot, along with the sugar and salt.

2 Place the pot on the stove and bring it to a boil. Once boiling, give it an immediate stir, cover the pot, and reduce the heat to low. Allow the rice to cook until all the liquid has been absorbed, which should take approximately 25 minutes. Remove the pot from the heat, fluff the rice with a fork, and keep it covered until you are ready to serve.

3 Before serving,the toasted coconut flakes should be stirred in gently.

6.4 YANGZHOU FRIED RICE

There is an abundant array of ingredients found in Yangzhou Fried Rice, also known as House or Special Fried Rice in local Chinese restaurants.

The primary ingredients typically consist of pork, shrimp, vegetables, and eggs. However, traditional versions may also incorporate chicken, sea cucumber, bamboo shoots, and scallops.

The name "Yangzhou Fried Rice" originates from the city of Yangzhou in Jiangsu province, China. Legend has it that sailors in Yangzhou would combine leftover lunch scraps to create a flavorful fried rice dish for dinner.

There are alternative claims suggesting that the dish actually originated in Guangzhou. Regardless of its exact origins, this dish has gained worldwide popularity for its harmonious blend of colorful and delicious ingredients.
This recipe boasts great versatility and serves as an excellent solution for utilizing leftover ingredients whenever the need arises.

INGREDIENTS

1 6 cups cooked white rice
2 3 eggs
3 2 scallions chopped
4 ½ cup barbecued pork
5 ⅓ cup peas frozen or fresh
6 1.5 tbsps soy sauce
7 3 tbsps cooking oil Pepper salt
8 2 carrots diced

STEP BY STEP PROCEDURE

1 Begin by gathering all the necessary ingredients. In a bowl, beat the eggs and season them with salt to your taste. Next, separate the grains of refrigerated rice by breaking them up.

2 Heat a wok or large pan over medium-high heat and add oil, swirling it around to coat the surface. Once the oil is hot and smoking, add the carrots and peas. Remove the pan from the heat.

3 Return the wok to the heat and add one tablespoon of oil, swirling it to ensure the bottom is coated. Add the rice to the wok and cook for 1-2 minutes, stirring and tossing the grains.

4 Create a space in the middle of the wok and add the remaining tablespoon of oil. Pour the beaten eggs into the space and cook for a few seconds while stirring. Mix the eggs with the rice and continue cooking while stirring and tossing. Check that the eggs are slightly runny and mostly cooked before reducing the heat.

5 Gently add the slices of barbecued pork into your Yangzhou fried rice. Follow this by adding the peas and carrots. Stir these ingredients in the wok, ensuring they are well combined. Proceed to add soy sauce and pepper, and cook for a few minutes while continuously stirring and tossing. Lastly, turn off the heat and introduce the chopped scallions. Thoroughly mix everything together and serve the dish while warm!

6.5 BRAISED RICE WITH SPARERIBS

This incredibly simple recipe for Chinese pork rib rice bowl is ideal for those who prefer an effortless cooking experience.

When I find myself wanting to minimize my time spent in the kitchen, this dish becomes my secret weapon. All I need to do is combine the ingredients and seasoning sauce in the rice cooker, and then press the "cook" button. In this post, I will gladly share with you the steps I took to create this delightful dish.

For this recipe, I used baby back ribs, as they are tender, flavorful, and slightly meatier than spare ribs. During your grocery store visit, you can ask the butcher to cut the ribs into bite-sized pieces, measuring around 2-3 inches each.

In addition to the pork ribs, I included diced shiitake mushrooms and mixed vegetables to enhance the texture and flavor of the dish. Once I rinsed the white rice, I placed all the ingredients on top of it in the cooking bowl. To add a touch of fragrance, I also added ginger and scallions on the surface.

INGREDIENTS

1 1 cup jasmine rice
2 1 cup fresh mixed vegetables (diced carrots, green peas, corns, green beans etc.)
3 2 stalks green onion, cut the white roots into 3-inch pieces and thinly slice the green portion for garnish later
4 ¾ cup water
5 1 pound baby back ribs (ask the butcher to cut them into 2-inch pieces for you)
6 A few drops of sesame oil for dressing at the end
7 2-3 thin slices of ginger
8 3-4 shiitake mushrooms, diced (or use fresh white mushrooms)

Sauce:

1 2.5 tablespoons soy sauce
2 1 tablespoon oyster sauce/hoisin sauce
3 1 tablespoon sugar
4 1 tablespoon cooking wine
5 Blanched vegetables or a fried egg on top (an optional topping)

STEP BY STEP PROCEDURE

1 Begin by rinsing the jasmine rice with water, then drain it and transfer it to the cooking bowl of a rice cooker.

2 In a small bowl, combine soy sauce, cooking wine, oyster sauce, and sugar. Mix thoroughly the ingredients and then place the bowl aside.

3 Heat a tablespoon of oil in a sauté pan over low heat, and sauté the pork ribs until they are slightly browned.

4 Add the cooked pork ribs, mushrooms, and mixed vegetables into the cooking bowl, placing them on top of the rice.

5 Arrange slices of ginger and green onion on the ingredients in the bowl, and then pour the seasoning sauce over them.

6 Add water to the bowl and gently stir everything with the rice spatula (provided with the rice cooker) to ensure the seasonings are well mixed.

7 Move the cooking bowl into the rice cooker, cover it with the lid, and press the "cook" button.

8 Once the rice is cooking, refrain from lifting the lid and allow it to cook undisturbed. After the rice cooker switches to the "keep warm" setting, let it sit for approximately 5 minutes.

9 With caution, remove the lid and use the rice spatula to transfer everything from the cooking bowl to a large plate or bowl.

10 Discard the ginger slices and green onion. Sprinkle the dish with chopped green onion and drizzle a small amount of sesame oil on top. Serve and savor the delicious flavors!

CHAPTER 7

APPETISERS/ STARTERS

Set aside the takeout menu and grab your kitchen tools. Homemade Chinese appetizers surpass the ones ordered from your beloved restaurant, and you'll relish the gratification of informing your guests that you prepared them from scratch. Whether it's egg rolls, dumplings, or lettuce wraps, these Chinese-inspired starters are ideal for any gathering, regardless of the theme.

A few of these recipes blend Asian and non-Asian elements, while others stay true to traditional Chinese cuisine. Once you've mastered the techniques, don't hesitate to add your personal touch to cater to your audience's preferences. Why rely on takeout when you can easily recreate your favourite popular Chinese appetizers in the comfort of your own home? Let's get started!

7.1. Vegetable Spring Rolls
7.2. Chinese style spareribs
7.3. Fried Shrimp Balls
7.4. Chinese Pork Pot Stickers
7.5. Baked Chicken Wonton
7.6. Lotus Leaf Wraps

7.1 VEGETABLE SPRING ROLLS

Preparing this vegetable-stuffed Chinese spring roll appetizer is simpler than you might imagine. By using vegetarian oyster sauce made from mushrooms, you can effortlessly transform these rolls into a vegan-friendly option.

Ever wondered about the origin of spring rolls? This light yet satisfying appetizer traces its roots back to the Chinese Spring Festival. Initially, spring rolls consisted of freshly harvested vegetables, with meat being incorporated at a later stage

INGREDIENTS

1 spring roll sheets, 1 packet
2 1/2 Chinese cabbage , cut into fine chiffonade
3 1 tbsp of coriander
4 1 tbsp of soy sauce
5 1/2 large carrot , cut into matchsticks

6 3 tsp cornflour, mixed with 3 tablespoons of water
7 1 tbsp of sesame oil
8 2 garlic cloves , minced
9 1 handful of bean sprouts
10 ginger , 2cm piece, minced
11 50g of rice noodles , vermicelli, broken into small pieces
12 1 tbsp of sesame oil
13 1 tbsp of rice wine, preferably shaoxing
14 salt
15 oil, for frying

STEP BY STEP PROCEDURE

1 Start by placing the noodles in warm water and allowing them to soak for 8-10 minutes.

2 Take a wok and heat it over high heat, adding sesame oil. Once hot, add cabbage, carrots, and beansprouts. Stir continuously and cook for 1 minute.

3 Introduce garlic and ginger into the wok and continue cooking for a few minutes until they become soft. Then, add soy sauce, shaoxing wine, spring onions, and coriander, stirring everything together.

4 Transfer the mixture to a bowl, allowing it to cool slightly while draining any excess moisture. Meanwhile, ensure the soaked noodles are well drained before adding them to the vegetable mixture.

5 To assemble the spring rolls, place a sheet of spring roll pastry on a clean work surface, positioning one corner towards you.

6 Take a tablespoon of the vegetable mixture and place it on the corner of the pastry. Roll the pastry tightly in a diagonal direction around the filling. Once you reach the middle of the pastry, fold in the corners from both sides. Brush a small amount of the cornflour mixture onto the remaining corner, then continue rolling up and press to seal.

7 Repeat the process with the remaining vegetable mixture and pastry sheets.

8 Heat a deep saucepan and fill it with oil, bringing it to a temperature of 180°C. Fry the spring rolls in batches for 2-3 minutes, or until they turn golden brown and become crispy. Serve the spring rolls immediately.

7.2. CHINESE STYLE SPARERIBS

Prepare these mouthwatering pork spareribs by baking them in the oven and coating them with a delightful honey and garlic sauce. This straightforward method yields incredible results.

Picnic salads like potato salad or coleslaw, along with cornbread muffins or hot buttered biscuits, make for excellent accompaniments to these delectable pork ribs. If you want to elevate the meal, consider serving twice-baked potatoes, or keep it simple with slow-cooked baked beans.

Quench your thirst with a refreshing glass of Southern iced tea with lemon or your favorite beer. Just remember to have plenty of napkins on hand for a satisfying eating experience.

INGREDIENTS

1 1/4 teaspoon freshly ground black pepper
2 1/4 cup soy sauce
3 4 pounds pork spareribs
4 3 tablespoons apple cider vinegar
5 1/4 teaspoon kosher salt
6 3 cloves garlic, finely minced
7 1/2 cup honey
8 1/4 teaspoon garlic powder

STEP BY STEP PROCEDURE

1 Gather all the necessary ingredients.

2 Preheat your oven to 325°F (165°C / Gas Mark 3) and line a large baking pan or roasting pan with foil.

3 If it's not yet done, gently remove the membrane/silverskin from the bone. You can get that done by sliding a narrow metal spatula possibly under the skin from one end.

4 Once the skin is loosened, grip it firmly with something like a cloth towel to aid firm grip and then pull the skin. It can actually come off all in one piece. But if that doesn't happen, then try to pull it again after using the knife to loosen the other end.

5 Cut the ribs into individual 1-rib pieces or portions suitable for serving.

6 Next, season the spare ribs with garlic powder, salt and then pepper.

7 Place the ribs in the prepared baking pan, arranging them evenly.

8 You can then cover the pan (let it be tightly covered), and bake for like an hour or until tender in the oven that you've preheated.

9 Once cooked, carefully drain off any excess fat and liquids from the pan.

10 Combine the garlic, vinegar, honey, including the soy sauce in a saucepan. Let it reach the boiling point.

11 Next, decrease the heat and allow to simmer for about 5-7 minutes.

12 Now, take up the temperature of the oven. You can increase it to about 180°C. Then, brush the garlic sauce and honey mixture over the spare ribs.

13 Keep baking the ribs for like 20-30 minutes (ensure it's uncovered), while you keep turning it until it's done. Once done, you can sieve and enjoy!

7.3 FRIED SHRIMP BALLS

These delectable Chinese shrimp balls are a delightful appetizer choice. Seasoned to perfection and featuring crispy water chestnuts, they are bound to impress your guests, whether served on an appetizer buffet or passed around. Feel free to select the ideal dipping sauce to accompany them, such as sweet and sour sauce, cocktail sauce, or spicy Chinese mustard sauce. A great advantage of this recipe is its flexibility to be prepared gluten-free by using gluten-free soy sauce and cornstarch.

INGREDIENTS

1 1 lb. shelled and deveined shrimp, defrost
2 1 teaspoon salt or fish sauce
3 1 teaspoon sugar
4 1 tablespoon oil or some pork fat
5 1 tablespoon corn starch
6 1/2 teaspoon sesame oil
7 1 egg white (slightly beaten)
8 8 pieces spring roll wrapper (8-inch square)
9 3 dashes white pepper powder

STEP BY STEP PROCEDURE

1 Place the shrimp, egg white, salt or fish sauce, sugar, cornstarch, sesame oil, regular oil, and white pepper in a mini food processor. Blend the ingredients until they form a smooth shrimp paste.

2 Take the spring roll wrappers and fold them up. Use a pair of scissors to cut the wrappers into small strips. Then, cut the strips into shorter pieces. After that, lay the strips on a flat surface. Moisten your hands and shape the shrimp paste into balls, using about 1 tablespoon of paste for each ball. Roll the shrimp balls over the bed of spring roll strips, ensuring they are coated.

3 Heat a deep fryer or a wok with oil. Deep fry the shrimp balls until they turn golden brown, which should take about 5 minutes. Remove the fried balls from the oil, allowing them to drain on paper towels. Serve the shrimp balls hot with Thai sweet chilli sauce or your preferred chilli sauce.

7.4 CHINESE PORK POT STICKERS

Trust me when I tell you that these homemade pork potstickers surpass any takeout option! Packed with succulent pork and cabbage, these potstickers boast the signature golden brown crispy bottoms.

Crafting pork and cabbage potstickers is not as daunting as it may seem. Once you experience the satisfaction of preparing these delectable dumplings at home, you'll find yourself wanting to make them time and time again. There's nothing quite like sinking your teeth into a dumpling with a juicy filling and perfectly crisp bottoms.

The filling for these pork potstickers features a savory blend of bok choy or napa cabbage, ground pork, and green onions, enhanced by a handful of simple yet flavorful ingredients. The result is a taste that rivals even the best frozen or restaurant potstickers. This recipe also includes instructions for preparing the dough and a basic dipping sauce to complement the dumplings.

INGREDIENTS

For the Filling:

1 8 ounces napa cabbage, or bok choy, about 1/2 large head
2 1 teaspoon cornstarch
3 1/4 cup finely chopped green onions, with tops
4 1 dash freshly ground white pepper
5 3 teaspoons salt, divided
6 1 pound lean ground pork
7 1 tablespoon white wine
8 1 teaspoon sesame oil

For the Dipping Sauce:

1 1 teaspoon sesame oil
2 1/4 cup soy sauce

For the Dumpling Dough:

1 1 cup of boiling water
2 2 cups all-purpose flour, plus more for working with dough

For Pan-Frying:

1 2 cups water, divided
2 2-4 tablespoons of vegetable oil

STEP BY STEP PROCEDURE

1 Collect together all the necessary ingredients.

2 Slice the bok choy or cabbage into thin strips and combine with 2 teaspoons of salt. Leave for like 5 minutes.

3 Squeeze out any excess moisture from the cabbage.

4 In a large bowl, mix together the cabbage, pork, green onions, wine, cornstarch, remaining 1 teaspoon of salt, sesame oil, and white pepper.

5 In a separate bowl, combine the flour and 1 cup of boiling water, stirring until a soft dough forms

6 Transfer the dough onto a lightly floured surface and knead for approximately 5 minutes, or until it becomes smooth.

7 Divide the dough in half. Shape each half into a 12-inch-long roll and cut each roll into 1/2-inch-thick slices.

8 Take one slice of dough and roll it into a 3-inch circle. Place approximately 1 tablespoon of the pork mixture in the centre of the circle.

9 Lift the edges of the circle and pinch them together, creating 5 pleats to form a pouch that encases the filling. Pinch the top to seal it.

10 Repeat the process with the remaining slices of dough and filling.

11 Heat a wok or nonstick skillet over medium-high heat until it becomes very hot. Add 1 tablespoon of vegetable oil, tilting the wok to ensure the sides are coated. If using a nonstick skillet, add 1/2 tablespoon of vegetable oil.

12 Place 12 dumplings in a single layer in the wok and fry them for approximately 2 minutes, or until the bottoms turn golden brown.

13 Pour 1/2 cup of water into the wok, cover it, and cook for 6 to 7 minutes, or until the water is absorbed.

14 Repeat the process with the remaining dumplings, using 1/2 to 1 tablespoon of vegetable oil and 1/2 cup of water for each batch.

15 For the dipping sauce, combine the soy sauce and 1 teaspoon of sesame oil in a small bowl.

16 Serve the flavorful dipping sauce alongside the dumplings. Enjoy your meal!

7.5 BAKED CHICKEN WONTON

Baked Chicken Wontons offer a healthier twist on the traditional cream cheese wontons. These delightful appetizers feature a chicken filling infused with the flavors of sesame, green onions, and sriracha.

This sumptuous chicken wonton recipe bakes instead of deep-frying the filled wontons. In addition, it makes use of reduced-fat peanut butter and a sugar substitute. If perhaps you're hosting a gathering/get-together of some sort, your health-conscious and weight-watching guests can savour these wontons without worrying about their waistlines.

You can also serve the wontons as a meal or appetiser, whichever suits you. While they're already bursting with flavor, you can enhance the experience by pairing them with a dipping sauce for example soy sauce, ketchup, sweet chili sauce, spicy Chinese mustard or cocktail sauce.

INGREDIENTS

1 1/2 pound chicken tenders approximately 5
2 6 ounces cream cheese room temperature
3 2 cloves garlic minced
4 1 teaspoon sriracha
5 1-2 tablespoons minced shallots or yellow onion finely diced
6 salt and pepper to taste
7 2 green onions thinly sliced
8 2 teaspoons soy sauce
9 Cooking Spray (like PAM)
10 1 teaspoon sesame oil
11 20 2- inch wonton wrappers
12 1 large egg beaten

STEP BY STEP PROCEDURE

1 Coat a medium skillet with PAM Cooking Spray and add the chicken. Add seasonings (pepper and salt) to your taste.

2 Place the skillet over medium-high heat and cook the chicken for 2 to 3 minutes. Spray the skillet with PAM Cooking Spray again and flip the chicken. Continue turning the chicken every 2 to 3 minutes until it is fully cooked and turns a golden brown color. This process should take around 6 to 8 minutes. Get the chicken from the skillet and then allow to cool. Once cooled, roughly chop the chicken
and set it aside.

3 In a medium mixing bowl, combine the cream cheese, shallots, garlic, green onions, soy sauce, sesame oil, and sriracha. Then, add the chopped chicken to the cream cheese mixture and keep stirring until well combined. Season with salt and pepper according to your preference.

4 Preheat the oven to 400 degrees F. Lightly oil a large baking sheet using PAM Cooking Spray. In a small bowl, whisk together the egg and 1 teaspoon of water until frothy, then set it aside.

5 Put together the wontons: Place the wrappers on your work surface and spoon less than or equal to 1 tablespoon of the cream cheese mixture into the centre of each wrapper. Use your

fingers to rub the edges of the wrappers with the egg and water mixture. Bring up two opposite sides of the wrapper and pinch them in the center, then bring up the remaining two sides to create an "X" shape and seal all the edges by pinching them together. Place the assembled wontons on the prepared baking sheet and repeat the process with the remaining wrappers and filling.

6 Arrange the wontons in a single layer on the baking sheet and place it in the preheated oven. Bake for 8 to 10 minutes, or until the wontons turn golden brown and crisp. Note: Check them around the 4 to 5-minute mark to avoid overcooking.

7 Serve the baked wontons immediately and enjoy!

Note that the cooking time for the chicken may vary depending on the thickness of your chicken slices or tenders.

7.6 LOTUS LEAF WRAPS

The delicate aroma of lotus leaves infuses these beautiful parcels with a subtle earthy flavor. The filling is absolutely delightful, and the sticky rice offers a satisfying chewiness. It all comes together to create a truly remarkable meal. To save on preparation time, you can make the filling ahead of time. If you're unable to find lotus leaves, you can easily substitute them with parchment paper.

INGREDIENTS

1 4 dried lotus leaves, halved
2 6 dried Chinese black mushrooms
3 6 ounces boneless, skinless chicken breast
4 2 cups glutinous rice (sticky rice is preferable)
5 1/4 teaspoon sesame oil
6 1 tablespoon light soy sauce
7 2 tablespoons Chinese rice wine, or dry sherry, divided
8 2 Chinese sausages (lap cheong)
9 1 clove garlic, finely chopped
10 1 teaspoon dark soy sauce
11 2 1/2 teaspoons cornstarch, divided
12 2 tablespoons vegetable oil
13 Freshly ground black or white pepper, to taste
14 Salt, to taste

STEP BY STEP PROCEDURE

1 Gather all the necessary ingredients.

2 Begin by soaking the lotus leaves in hot water for approximately 1 hour.

3 Place the rice in a bowl and cover it with water. Allow the rice to soak for 1 hour.

4 After the soaking time, gently pat the lotus leaves dry and drain the rice.

5 Steam the rice using a bamboo steamer lined with parchment paper. Fill a wok halfway with water and bring it to a boil. Place the steamer on top of the wok, ensuring it doesn't touch the water. Spread the drained rice evenly in the steamer, cover it, and steam for about 25 minutes or until the rice becomes tender. Once cooked, keep the rice covered and warm while you prepare the remaining ingredients.

6 In the meantime, soften the dried mushrooms by soaking them in hot water for approximately 20 to 30 minutes.

7 Squeeze out any excess water from the mushrooms and finely chop them, discarding any tough stems if necessary.

8 Cut the chicken into small cubes, approximately 1/2 inch in size.

9 In a medium bowl, combine salt, 1 tablespoon rice wine, and 1 teaspoon cornstarch. Mix well. Add the chicken pieces and let them marinate at room temperature for 20 minutes.

10 If desired, remove the casings from the sausage. Finely slice or chop the sausages. Peel and chop the garlic.

11 In a small bowl, combine the remaining 1 tablespoon rice wine, light soy sauce, and dark soy sauce. In another small bowl, dissolve the remaining 1 1/2 teaspoons cornstarch in 1 tablespoon of water. Whisk the cornstarch mixture into the rice wine-soy sauce mixture.

12 Heat a wok over medium-high heat and add the vegetable oil. Once the oil shimmers, add the garlic and stir-fry for about 30 seconds until fragrant. Add the marinated chicken and stir-fry until it turns opaque and is mostly cooked through, approximately 3 minutes.

13 Add the sausages and mushrooms to the wok. Stir-fry for 1 minute. Give the sauce mixture a quick stir, then add it to the center of the wok. Stir quickly until the sauce thickens. Season with pepper to taste. Continue to cook, stirring everything together until heated through, for 1 to 2 minutes. Remove from heat and stir in the sesame oil. Allow the mixture to cool.

14 To assemble the wraps, divide the rice and filling into 8 equal portions (1 portion for each wrap). Place a lotus leaf, right side down, on a work surface. Using damp hands, gently flatten one-half portion of rice into a round disk, approximately 3 1/2 inches wide. Place the rice in the center of the lotus leaf. Top the rice with one portion of the filling, shaping the rice with your hands to form a ring around the filling. Add the remaining one-half portion of rice to cover the filling.

15 Create a square parcel by folding the lotus leaf over the filling, ensuring that the filling is completely covered. Secure the package with kitchen twine. Repeat the process with the remaining rice, filling, and lotus leaves.

16 Steam the lotus leaf parcels in a covered bamboo steamer placed in a wok. You can also make use of a Vegetable Steamer. Steam the parcels for approximately 15 minutes, until they are hot and the chicken is fully cooked.

17 To serve, remove and discard the twine. Unwrap the parcels, folding the lotus leaves down around the filling (you do not have to eat the leaves). Enjoy!

CHAPTER 8

EGGS AND POULTRY

Chinese cuisine has gained tremendous popularity worldwide, permeating every nook and cranny. With an extensive array of recipes catering to diverse dietary preferences, taste buds, and meal occasions, it's no surprise that we simply can't resist!

While Chinese dishes are typically celebrated for their meat, vegetables, and rice, eggs play an equally crucial role in elevating classic recipes. Not only do eggs impart a delightful flavor, but they also offer vital nutrients. Depending on the cooking method employed, eggs can enhance both the texture and taste of a dish, serving as the primary protein source or a delightful complement.

Let's check out some of the types of egg recipes:

8.1. Chinese Egg Tarts
8.2. Chow Mein
8.3. Chinese Egg Foo Yung
8.4. Chinese Egg Fried Rice
8.5. Cantonese Scrambled Egg
8.6. Chinese Steamed Egg
8.7. Chinese Tea Eggs
8.8. Chinese Egg Drop Soup

8.1 CHINESE EGG TARTS

If you're a fan of Cantonese dim sum, chances are you're well-acquainted with the delectable Hong Kong egg tarts. While barbecue meat buns may steal the spotlight as the quintessential item in dim sum restaurants and Chinese bakeries, the most adored dessert undoubtedly goes to the Hong Kong egg tart. These delightful treats trace their origins back to the Portuguese pastel de nata, introduced to Macau when the Portuguese first arrived in the early 20th century.

INGREDIENTS

Oil dough
1 200 g plain flour

2 325 g butter

Water dough
1 250 g plain flour
2 100 g of ice water
3 1/2 teaspoon of salt
4 1 egg

Filling:
1 5 eggs
2 165 ml of water
3 80 ml milk
4 Egg tart molds
5 80 g caster sugar

STEP BY STEP PROCEDURE

1 Water Dough: In an electric food processor, combine plain flour, egg, and ice water.

2 Mix the ingredients until they form a cohesive ball.

3 Oil Dough: Cut chilled butter into small pieces.

4 Add the butter and flour to the electric food processor.

5 Use the pulse function to mix them until the mixture forms bridges and strands, resembling a crumbly texture.

Chinese Puff Pastry Preparation:
6 Place a large piece of cling film on the tabletop and sprinkle it with plain flour.

7 Flatten the water dough and place another piece of cling film on top.

8 Roll out the water dough to form a large square.

9 Remove the cling film from the top of the water dough and place the oil dough in the centre. Fold the sides of the water dough over the oil dough, ensuring the oil dough is completely covered by the water dough.

10 Flatten it with a rolling pin. (Analogy: The dough resembles a sandwich, with the oil dough as the filling and the water dough as the bread.)

11 Wrap the dough in cling film and refrigerate for twenty minutes or until it becomes firm.

12 Remove the dough from the refrigerator and flatten it with a rolling pin to approximately 3cm thickness. Fold both ends of the dough towards the center, similar to closing a book. (Analogy: It now resembles a multilayered sandwich.) Place it in the refrigerator again for 20 minutes.

13 Repeat the folding process (step 6) three more times.

14 After the final repetition, roll out the dough to approximately 3 mm thickness.

15 Use a cookie cutter or a bowl to cut out round pastry pieces slightly larger than the size of the molds.

16 Place the cut pastry into the molds and lightly press it onto the surface.

17 Trim the edges with a fork or a blunt knife.

8.2 CHOW MEIN

Indulge in the timeless Chinese delight of stir-fried egg noodles featuring tender shredded chicken breast. Feel free to explore variations with different fish, meat, or vegetables, adding your own creative touch.

These noodles hold a cherished place in Chinese culinary traditions, with the oldest known recipe tracing back centuries. Typically crafted from eggs and either wheat or rice flour, making egg noodles from scratch is a simple yet rewarding process. However, if you prefer convenience, store-bought noodles can be used as well.

To bring this dish to life, gather a remarkable ensemble of ingredients: chow mein egg noodles, oil, garlic, chicken, shrimp, cabbage, carrots, and scallions. For the delightful sauce, you'll need light and dark soy sauce, oyster sauce, sugar, and water.

INGREDIENTS

1 8 oz. steamed chow mein or fresh chow mein noodles

Chow Mein Sauce:

1 1 tablespoon soy sauce
2 1/2 teaspoon dark soy sauce
3 1/2 teaspoon sugar
4 2 tablespoons water
5 1 tablespoon oyster sauce

Other Ingredients:

1 1/4 cup shredded carrot
2 2 oz. chicken, (they should be cut into thin strips)
3 6 medium-sized shrimp (shelled and deveined)
4 3 cloves garlic (finely minced)
5 1/2 cup shredded cabbage
6 2 tablespoons cooking oil
7 2 stalks scallions (cut into 2-inch strips (5 cm))

STEP BY STEP PROCEDURE

1 Begin by soaking the chow mein noodles in cold water for approximately 5 minutes. Rinse them a few times until the water runs clear and the noodles become soft. Drain off any excess water and set the noodles aside. (Avoid over-soaking, as it may result in soggy noodles.)

2 In a small mixing bowl, combine all the ingredients for the Chow Mein Sauce. Mix well and set the sauce aside.

3 Heat a skillet or wok with oil over
medium heat. Add the garlic and stir-fry until it turns light brown and releases its aromatic fragrance. Add the chicken and shrimp, stir-frying until they are halfway cooked. Toss in the shredded cabbage and carrot, giving them a quick stir-fry. Introduce the soaked noodles and the prepared soy sauce mixture to the wok. Continue stir-frying until the noodles are thoroughly coated with the sauce and fully cooked.

4 Sprinkle in the chopped scallions, give it a final few stirs, and then transfer the dish to a serving plate. Serve hot and enjoy!

8.3 CHINESE EGG FOO YUNG

Egg foo yung, also known as egg foo young, is a cherished dish that can be found in Chinese and British American restaurants, as well as in Chinese Indonesian cuisine. Resembling a pancake-omelet, this delightful creation combines eggs with various proteins, vegetables, and flavors, resulting in a savory treat. Unlike a traditional omelet, egg foo yung is pan-fried until it reaches a golden brown color, which sets it apart. While commonly filled with shrimp or pork and an assortment of vegetables, the possibilities for variations are endless, allowing each cook to put their unique spin on the dish. It's a versatile recipe that welcomes the use of leftovers, making it an ideal choice. You can get creative and include your favorite ingredients to personalize your own version of egg foo yung. To enhance the meal, a savory and umami-flavored gravy accompanies it, making it suitable for breakfast-for-dinner or any time of the day. It's a satisfying and straightforward recipe, and you can add all your preferred veggies to it. For a wholesome and well-rounded meal, serve it with rice. Before you begin, make sure to acquire lap cheong, a Chinese sausage readily available online or at Asian markets.

INGREDIENTS

For the Sauce:

1 1/2 cup low-sodium chicken broth
2 Freshly ground black pepper, or white pepper, to taste
3 1 tablespoon Chinese rice wine, or dry sherry
4 1 dash sesame oil

5 1 tablespoon light soy sauce
6 1 teaspoon cornstarch
7 6 teaspoons water

For the Egg Foo Yung:

1 5 large eggs
2 Freshly ground black pepper, to taste
3 2 to 3 teaspoons Chinese rice wine, or dry sherry
4 6 mushrooms, sliced
5 1/2 cup napa cabbage, thinly sliced
6 1 teaspoon kosher salt, or more to taste
7 3 tablespoons canola oil, divided
8 3 Chinese sausages, sliced into 1/4-inch pieces
9 1/4 cup chopped onion
10 1/2 cup mung bean sprouts

For Serving:

1 4 cups steamed rice
2 3 green onions, sliced (this is optional though).

STEP BY STEP PROCEDURE

1 Preparing the Sauce: Collect all the necessary ingredients.

2 Place the chicken broth in a saucepan and bring it to a boil over medium heat. Stir in the soy sauce, rice wine, sesame oil, and season with pepper to taste. Slightly increase the heat and add the cornstarch dissolved in water, stirring quickly to thicken the sauce.

3 Move the saucepan to a different burner and keep the sauce warm on low heat while you proceed to make the egg foo yung omelette.

Making the Egg Foo Yung Omelet:

4 Gather all the required ingredients.

5 In a medium bowl, lightly beat the eggs. Add pepper, rice wine, and salt to the beaten eggs. Set the egg mixture aside.

6 Heat 1 tablespoon of oil in a frying pan over medium heat. Once the oil is hot, add the onion and sausage. Stir-fry for about 2 minutes, then remove them from the pan using a slotted spoon and set them aside.

7 Add another tablespoon of oil to the pan and stir-fry the sliced mushrooms until they turn brown. Get then off the pan and put aside.

8 Add the cooked sausages, onion, mushrooms, mung bean sprouts, and napa cabbage to the egg mixture.

9 Add the remaining tablespoon of oil to the pan. Once the oil is hot, pour in the egg mixture. Cook the omelet until the bottom side turns golden brown.

10 Carefully flip the omelet over and cook the other side until it also becomes golden brown.

11 Serve the egg foo yung omelet hot, with the warmed sauce poured over the top. If desired, garnish with green onions. Accompany it with steamed rice for a delightful meal. Enjoy!

8.4 CHINESE EGG FRIED RICE

This egg fried rice recipe holds a special place in my heart as one of my favorite side dishes, especially when I'm cooking up a Chinese feast. In fact, it's versatile enough to serve as a satisfying main course too.

There's something truly comforting about homemade fried rice. It not only fills you up but also provides essential vitamins and nutrients. Amongst the various fried rice variations, egg fried rice stands out, elevating your fried rice experience to new heights. The key to achieving incredible fried rice lies in using day-old rice. Allowing the rice to dry out and firm up overnight ensures that the grains remain separate and firm during the frying process, preventing mushy rice.

What makes this dish even more appealing is its adaptability. It's perfect for picky eaters as you can easily substitute the ingredients with your preferred vegetables or meats. Feel free to personalize it according to your taste and cravings.

INGREDIENTS

1 1 onion, finely chopped
2 2 eggs, beaten
3 1 tbsp rapeseed (canola) oil
4 3 cloves garlic, finely chopped
5 800g (4 cups) cooked Jasmine or long grain rice
6 ½ tsp ground white pepper
7 2 tbsp soy sauce or more to taste
8 1 tbsp lemon juice
9 2 tbsp sesame oil
10 4 spring onions (scallions) thinly sliced

STEP BY STEP PROCEDURE

1 Heat 2 tablespoons of oil in a wok over high heat. Add the chopped onions and stir-fry for approximately 3 minutes until they begin to soften. Next, add the chopped garlic and continue frying for an additional 30 seconds.

2 Introduce the cooked rice to the wok and drizzle with sesame oil. Stir-fry the rice, ensuring it is thoroughly coated with the oil and heated through.

3 Push the rice to one side of the wok and pour in the beaten eggs and soy sauce. Stir the eggs gently to scramble them, then incorporate them into the rice mixture.

4 Using a spoon or spatula, gently push the rice around in the wok, rather than stirring it vigorously. This helps distribute the flavours without breaking the rice grains.

5 Taste the fried rice and adjust the seasoning by adding more soy sauce if desired, to achieve a richer savory flavor.

6 Squeeze in lemon juice according to your taste preferences. Adjust the amount as desired.

7 Serve the egg fried rice immediately, garnished with chopped spring onions for an extra burst of freshness.

8.5 CANTONESE SCRAMBLED EGGS

Cantonese Scrambled Eggs is a popular and beloved dish that has gained widespread popularity worldwide. It is enjoyed by millions of people every day. Not only is it simple and quick to make, but it also boasts a delightful and delicious flavor. Cantonese Scrambled Eggs has been a personal favorite of mine for as long as I can remember. These eggs are not only delicious, but they also have an appealing visual appeal. It's not just a Chinese dish; it's a truly scrumptious culinary experience that anyone can enjoy.

INGREDIENTS

1 5 Large eggs
2 1/2 tsp salt
3 1 tsp cornstarch
4 1/2 tsp sesame oil
5 1 tbsp ghee or lard
6 1/2 tsp Shaoxing or Rice wine
7 1/8 tsp (Pinch) white pepper powder
8 1/8 tsp (Pinch) MSG
9 1/2 tsp sugar
10 1 tbsp water

STEP BY STEP PROCEDURE

1 Prepare a slurry by combining cornstarch and water.

2 In a bowl, mix together salt, sugar, wine, sesame oil, pepper, and MSG.

3 Separate the egg whites from the yolks. Whisk the egg whites until they become bubbly. Combine the egg whites with the yolks and whisk briefly until well mixed.

4 Add the seasoning mixture and cornstarch slurry to the eggs. Whisk briefly to incorporate all the ingredients.

5 Heat a coated pan and pour in the egg mixture. Utilize a cooking technique where you pull away the cooked portion of the eggs and allow the uncooked portion to gather on the hot side of the pan. This creates a layered effect. Be careful not to overcook the eggs; they should remain moist.

Optional: Enhance the dish by adding your favorite protein, such as green onions or scallions, bean sprouts, cheese, or any other desired ingredients.

8.6 CHINESE STEAMED EGG

Chinese Steamed Egg, also known as Chinese Steamed Egg Custard, is a nutritious breakfast option. It is a traditional dish that can be found throughout China, even with the vast regional differences in cuisine. Despite its simple ingredients of eggs and water, this recipe yields a delicately flavored and silky smooth texture. Don't be fooled by its basic components; the Chinese Steamed Egg offers a delightful and velvety experience for your taste buds.

INGREDIENTS

1 4 medium-sized eggs
2 1 pinch salt (this is optional)
3 1 ¼ - 1 ¾ cups water, vegetable, or chicken stock (approximately, as it will depend on the volume of your eggs) - lightly warmed

FOR THE TOPPINGS
1 sesame oil
2 chives - finely chopped
3 hot chilli oil
4 soy sauce (use tamari for GF)

STEP BY STEP PROCEDURE

DETERMINE THE AMOUNT OF STOCK OR WATER NEEDED

1 Start by determining the quantity of water or stock required. Since egg sizes can vary, it's best to measure the volume of the eggs you are using for this recipe. In a medium bowl, lightly beat the eggs with a fork. Take note of the volume (in cups or milliliters). If you have a 2-cup measuring cup, you can beat the eggs directly into it to obtain a measurement. For example, my four eggs amounted to 200 milliliters (just under 1 cup).

2 The amount of water or stock needed should be approximately 1 ½ to 2 times the volume of the eggs. So, if you have 200 milliliters of eggs, you can use between 300 to 400 milliliters of water, depending on your preference. Using 300 milliliters will result in a firmer texture compared to using 400 milliliters.

PREPARE THE CHINESE STEAMED EGGS

3 Gradually pour the water into the beaten eggs. If desired, add salt to taste.

4 Pour the egg mixture through a fine mesh strainer, dividing it evenly into two bowls. The strainer will catch any larger pieces of egg and help remove bubbles or foam that may have formed. If time permits, let the mixture rest for a few minutes to allow any remaining bubbles on the surface to dissipate.

5 Cover the bowls with aluminum foil to prevent water droplets from the steamer falling directly onto the eggs, which could create a rough surface.

6 Place the bowls carefully in a prepared steamer. Steam over low heat until the eggs are set, typically around 10-14 minutes, depending on the shape and depth of the bowls.

7 Remove the bowls from the steamer with caution and garnish the steamed eggs with your preferred toppings. Serve the dish warm.

8.7 CHINESE TEA EGGS

Indulge in the delightful taste of Chinese tea eggs, the ultimate way to enjoy hard-boiled eggs! These eggs are not only bursting with flavor but also boast an exquisite marble appearance. They serve as a fantastic high-protein and low-calorie snack.
Tea eggs have a long-standing tradition and are beloved treats in China, Indonesia, and Taiwan. Although they require some time to prepare, the result is well worth it, as they can be enjoyed for up to three or four days. With this unique recipe, you can achieve perfectly tender tea eggs every single time.
Unlike ordinary hard-boiled eggs, tea eggs require a handful of additional ingredients to unlock an unrivaled flavor profile. Sichuan peppercorns, ginger, bay leaves, light and dark soy sauce, star anise, black tea leaves, sugar, salt, and a cinnamon stick come together to create a symphony of tastes that will tantalize your taste buds.

INGREDIENTS

1 8 eggs - at room temperature
2 2 bags black tea - or 1 tablespoon of loose tea
3 ½ teaspoon Sichuan peppercorn
4 1 star-anise
5 1 bay leaf
6 2 teaspoon salt
7 1 piece Chinese cinnamon - aka cassia cinnamon
8 2 tablespoon dark soy sauce

9 1 tablespoon light soy sauce
10 1 teaspoon Shaoxing rice wine - optional
11 ½ tablespoon sugar

STEP BY STEP PROCEDURE

1 Fill a pot or saucepan with plenty of water, making sure it's enough to cover all the eggs. Bring the water to a full boil. Carefully add the eggs to the boiling water and let them cook uncovered over medium heat for 8 minutes. If you prefer softer yolks, reduce the cooking time to 7 minutes.

2 While the eggs are cooking, take a clean saucepan and combine all the remaining ingredients. This includes the tea, spices, and seasonings. Add 2 cups (500ml) of water to the saucepan. Bring the mixture to a boil and let it simmer for 3 minutes. Set it aside.

3 Once the eggs are cooked, transfer them to a large bowl filled with cold water. Allow them to cool down until they are safe to handle. To create the beautiful marbled effect, gently crack the shells of each egg by lightly tapping them on the kitchen counter, ensuring that the shells are cracked all around.

4 Place the cracked eggs in a container, ideally one that can hold them snugly. Pour the prepared marinade over the eggs, ensuring they are fully submerged. Cover the container with a lid and let the eggs steep in the marinade for 12 to 24 hours before serving. This will infuse them with rich flavors.

5 If you have leftover marinade, you can reuse it for future batches. It's recommended to freeze the marinade if you don't plan on using it soon. When you're ready to use it again, simply add more tea, spices, and seasonings as needed. Remember to always bring the marinade to a boil before using it to prevent any bacterial growth.
Enjoy your homemade Chinese tea eggs, packed with flavor and boasting a beautiful marbled appearance!

8.8 CHINESE EGG DROP SOUP

The dish known as "Egg Drop" gets its name from the method of making the soup—dropping raw egg into hot broth. It's a simple concept that doesn't require a genius to understand.

Interestingly, the direct translation of this dish in Chinese is "egg flower soup," referring to the beautiful swirls created by the egg in the soup, resembling the pattern of a flower.
While there are numerous versions of egg drop soup, the recipe provided here is a classic rendition that mimics the restaurant-style preparation, allowing you to enjoy this delicious soup in the comfort of your own home.

INGREDIENTS

1 4 cups chicken stock (about 1 liter, organic or homemade preferred!)
2 3 tablespoons cornstarch (mixed with 1/3 cup water)

3 3/4 teaspoon salt
4 1/4 teaspoon MSG (you can increase it as you prefer)
5 1/2 teaspoon sesame oil
6;1/8 teaspoon white pepper
7 1/2 teaspoon turmeric (Or 5 drops yellow food coloring. This is optional though)
8 3 eggs (lightly beaten)
9 1 scallion (chopped)
10 1/8 teaspoon sugar.

STEP BY STEP PROCEDURE

1 Heat the chicken stock in a medium soup pot until it reaches a simmer. Add the sesame oil, salt, sugar, white pepper, and MSG (if desired). For an optional rich yellow color, you can include turmeric or a few drops of yellow food coloring. Taste the soup and season as you wish.

2 In a separate bowl, mix the cornstarch and water thoroughly to create a slurry. Ensure that the cornstarch is well incorporated as it tends to settle quickly. While stirring the soup continuously, gradually pour in the slurry to avoid any lumps of cooked starch. Adjust the amount of starch to achieve your desired soup consistency. If preferred, you can add the starch in small batches, simmering the soup in between to check the thickness.

3 Now comes the exciting part—adding the egg. Lightly beat the egg before incorporating it into the soup. The speed at which you stir the soup while adding the egg will determine the size of the egg swirls. To create large "egg flowers" or smaller swirly bits of egg, use a ladle to stir the soup in a circular motion while slowly drizzling in the beaten egg.

4 Serve the soup in bowls, garnish with chopped scallions, and enjoy!

CHAPTER 9

BEEF AND PORK

Pork holds a position of immense popularity in Chinese cuisine, reigning as the most widely consumed meat in the country. Let's consider some of them!

9.1. Char siu
9.2. Shabu-shabu
9.3. Crispy Fried Chicken
9.4. Kung Pao Chicken
9.5. Peking Duck
9.6. Orange Chicken

9.1 CHAR SIU

Char siu is a delectable dish comprised of succulent, barbecued pork that undergoes a prior marinade in the renowned char siu sauce. This flavorsome sauce incorporates ingredients like soy sauce, hoisin sauce, rice wine, and star anise. The pork is typically presented as either appetizing slices or shredded and chopped for a satisfying main course.

During the early stages of char siu's creation, various meats such as wild boars and pigs were utilized to prepare this dish. The term "char siu" directly translates to "fork-roasted," alluding to the original cooking technique of skewering the meat on an elongated fork and roasting it over an open fire. This process results in the delightful caramelization of the marinade's sugars.

INGREDIENTS

1 ½ teaspoon five spice powder
2 ¼ teaspoon white pepper
3 ½ teaspoon sesame oil
4 1/8 teaspoon red food colouring (this is optional though)
5 2 teaspoons salt

6 ¼ cup granulated white sugar

7 1 tablespoon Shaoxing rice wine

8 1 tablespoon soy sauce

9 2 teaspoons molasses

10 3 cloves finely minced garlic

11 2 tablespoons maltose or honey

12 1 tablespoon hot water

13 1 tablespoon hoisin sauce

14 3 pounds boneless pork shoulder/pork butt (you should select a piece with some good fat on it).

STEP BY STEP PROCEDURE

1 Slice or cut the pork into long strips or chunks, approximately 2 to 3 inches thick. Keep the excess fat intact as it will render off during cooking and enhance the flavor.

2 In a bowl, combine sugar, salt, five spice powder, white pepper, sesame oil, wine, soy sauce, hoisin sauce, molasses, food coloring (if desired), and garlic to create the marinade, also known as the BBQ sauce.

3 Take about 2-3 tablespoons of marinade and keep to use later. Then, gently rub the pork with the remaining marinade in a large bowl/baking dish. After this, cover the pork and pit in the fridge for 8 hours minimum. You should store the reserved marinade in the refrigerator as well.

4 Preheat your oven to 475°F. The setting should be on the 'bake'. Please take note that oven temperatures can vary, so then you can use an oven thermometer for accurate readings. Monitor the char siu every 10-15 minutes and adjust the temperature if necessary.

5 Place a metal rack ok top of a lined sheet pan. The essence of the rack is to ensure even roasting by keeping the pork elevated. Arrange the marinated pork on the rack, leaving sufficient space between the pieces. After them, pour 1 ½ cups of water into the pan beneath the rack to prevent any drippings from burning.

6 Then, place the sheet pan in the preheated oven. Roast for 25-30 minutes, maintaining the oven temperature at 475°F (246°C) for the first 10 minutes. Then, you can reduce the oven temperature to 375°F (190°C). After about 25 minutes, flip the pork over. If the bottom of the pan is dry, try to add another cup of water. You should also rotate the pan 180 degrees to make sure that they are roasted evenly. Keep roasting for an additional 15 minutes, checking regularly to prevent burning and adjusting the oven temperature if necessary.

7 While the pork is roasting, combine the reserved marinade with maltose or honey (if using maltose, you can warm it in the microwave for easier handling) and 1 tablespoon of hot water. This mixture will serve as the basting sauce for the pork.

8 After roasting for about 40 minutes, brush the pork with the basting sauce, flip it over, and baste the other side as well. Continue roasting for an additional 10 minutes.

9 At this point, the pork would have been roasted for a total of 50 minutes. It should be thoroughly cooked and caramelised on the surface. But if you desire further caramelization, you

can,.for a moment, turn on the broiler for like 2-4 minutes to crisp the outside and enhance the colour and flavour. Be cautious not to leave it unattended, as the sweet char siu BBQ sauce can burn quickly. In another way, you can use a meat thermometer to check if the internal temperature of the pork has reached 160°F (71°C).

10 Remove the pork from the oven and brush it with the remaining reserved BBQ sauce. Allow the meat to rest for 10 minutes before slicing. Finally, savor the flavors of your perfectly cooked char siu!

9.2 SHABU SHABU

Shabu shabu, a delightful hot pot recipe, originated in Osaka, Japan during the 1950s and quickly gained popularity throughout the country, drawing inspiration from Chinese hot pot traditions. The name "shabu shabu" (pronounced shah-boo shah-boo) derives from the onomatopoeic sound created when the ingredients are gently swished around in the simmering broth.

This dish holds a special place in our hearts as it is cherished both when prepared at home and enjoyed in restaurants. It exudes an air of elegance while being remarkably simple to assemble, offering a burst of flavors that never fails to impress.

One of the remarkable aspects of shabu shabu is that it falls under the category of nabemono, which translates to "things in one pot" in Japanese. This highlights the essence of communal dining, where various ingredients are cooked together in a shared pot, enhancing the sense of togetherness and enjoyment. The term "nabe" refers to the cooking pot, while "mono" signifies the collection of ingredients.

INGREDIENTS

1 8 cups water sub with homemade dashi stock
2 2 tsp dashi powder
3 ¼ cabbage chopped
4 3 spring onion / green onion sliced into lengths of 6cm / 1.5in
5 250 g udon noodles frozen
6 300 g firm tofu chopped
7 100 g enoki mushrooms broken into small bunches
8 200 g pork thinly sliced for hot pot
9 1 carrot diagonally sliced
10 6 shiitake mushrooms stalks removed

Dipping Sauces
1 4 tbsp ponzu
2 4 tbsp goma dare (Sesame Sauce)

STEP BY STEP PROCEDURE

1 In a medium saucepan, nabe pot, or electric frypan, bring 8 cups of water and 2 tsp of dashi powder to a boil over high heat.

2 While the water is heating up, prepare the vegetables for cooking. Cut the cabbage into approximately 3cm x 3cm (1.5 inch) squares, tofu into 2cm x 2cm (1 inch) squares, carrot diagonally sliced, spring onions into 6cm (2.5 inch) lengths, enoki mushrooms with the roots removed and separated into small bunches, and remove the stalks from the shiitake mushrooms. Place all the vegetables on one plate next to the shabu shabu pot.

3 Place the pork on another plate and position it alongside the vegetables. If using frozen udon noodles, loosen and thaw them by pouring boiling water over them in a bowl. Drain and transfer them to a separate bowl, placing it next to the meat and vegetables.

4 Prepare the dipping sauces by filling two small sauce bowls per person at the table. Fill one bowl with 2 tbsp of ponzu and the other with 2 tbsp of sesame sauce. Place them in front of each person along with a set of chopsticks or a fork if preferred.

5 If serving rice with your shabu shabu, prepare a small bowl for each person and place them in front of the dipping sauces.

6 You are now ready to commence your shabu shabu experience!

How to eat shabu shabu:
7. Once the dashi broth reaches a boil, reduce the heat to a simmer and begin the shabu shabu process

8 Start by adding carrot and cabbage to the simmering broth, as they require the longest cooking time (approximately 3 minutes). Then, add udon noodles, mushrooms, and tofu (which only need around 1 minute to cook). Add enough of each ingredient for everyone to have a portion, and avoid overcrowding the pot to prevent overcooking.

9 Now it's time to add the meat! Shabu shabu meat is thin and cooks quickly, usually requiring just about 30 seconds. Add a few slices at a time to avoid overcooking. The meat is ready to eat when it changes color from pink to a light brown.

10 When removing ingredients from the pot, use chopsticks or a slotted spoon. It's time to dip! Traditionally, meat is dipped in sesame sauce and vegetables in ponzu, but feel free to mix and match sauces according to your preference.

11 Once dipped, you can enjoy the ingredients directly or pair them with some rice. By the end of the meal, your rice bowl will be filled with delicious flavors from the soup and ingredients, so savor the combination.

9.3 CRISPY FRIED CHICKEN

When it comes to chicken, few things can compare to the sheer deliciousness of a succulent, crispy piece of finger-licking good fried chicken. The idea of frying your own chicken may seem daunting, but fear not, as it is a surprisingly simple process that surpasses the quality of store-bought and fast-food fried chicken by a long shot. With a reliable oil thermometer and a timer at your disposal, you can effortlessly create a batch of perfectly fried chicken every time. If you've ever had the desire to venture into the realm of homemade fried chicken, there's no better time than now to give it a try!

INSTRUCTIONS

1 1 (4 pound) chicken, cut into pieces
2 2 quarts vegetable oil for frying
3 2 cups all-purpose flour for coating
4 1 teaspoon paprika
5 1 cup buttermilk
6 salt and pepper to taste

STEP BY STEP PROCEDURE

1 Take your chicken pieces and, if desired, remove the skin.

2 Place the flour in a large plastic bag. The amount of flour should depend on the quantity of chicken you're cooking. Add seasonings (salt, pepper and paprika) to taste. Paprika helps in achieving a nicely browned chicken.

3 Dip the chicken pieces in buttermilk, then take a few at a time and place them inside the bag with the flour. Seal the bag and shake it well to coat the chicken evenly.

4 Transfer the coated chicken onto a cookie sheet or tray. Cover it with a clean dish towel or waxed paper. Allow the chicken to sit until the flour forms a paste-like consistency. This step is crucial for achieving the desired texture.

5 In a large skillet (preferably cast iron), pour vegetable oil to fill about 1/3 to 1/2 of the skillet's capacity. Heat the oil very hot.

6 Place as many chicken pieces as the skillet can hold without overcrowding. Brown the chicken on both sides in the hot oil.

7 Once the chicken is browned, reduce the heat and cover the skillet. Let the chicken cook for 30 minutes, ensuring it is cooked through but not yet crispy. Remove the cover, increase the heat, and continue frying until the chicken turns crispy.

8 Drain the fried chicken on paper towels to remove excess oil. Depending on the quantity of chicken, you may need to fry in batches. Keep the finished chicken warm by placing it in a slightly warm oven while you prepare the remaining batches.

9.4 KUNG PAO CHICKEN

Elevate your Kung Pao Chicken game by preparing it at home and surpassing the taste of Chinese takeout! Experience the perfect balance of tender, crispy chicken combined with a heavenly, velvety Chinese sauce that bursts with incredible flavors.

Traditionally, Kung Pao chicken is a dry-stir fry dish, with just the right amount of sauce to enhance the flavors. However, the explosion of flavors in this dish is so remarkable that you won't feel the need for additional sauce. The richness and depth of taste are truly extraordinary!

INGREDIENTS

 For the chicken:

1 28 ounces (800g) boneless/skinless
chicken breast (that is cut into 1 inch cubes)
2 1 teaspoon cornstarch / corn flour
3 1 tablespoon light soy sauce
4 2 teaspoons baking soda
5 1 tablespoon shaoxing wine or dry sherry

For the sauce:

1 1/2 cup low-sodium chicken stock (or broth) -- water can be used
2 2 teaspoon dark soy sauce
3 2 tablespoons Chinese black vinegar (or substitute good-quality balsamic vinegar)
4 2 tablespoon Chinese Shaoxing wine (or dry sherry)
5 2 tablespoons sugar
6;5 tablespoons light soy sauce
7 2 teaspoons hoisin sauce
8 1 teaspoon cornstarch / corn flour

For the stir fry:

1 4 tablespoons cooking oil divided
2 1 1/2 tablespoons garlic (4-6 cloves)
3 1/2 green bell pepper (capsicum) seeded and diced
4 4 green onion / scallion stems cut into 1-inch pieces
5 1/2 red bell pepper (capsicum) seeded and diced
6 1/2 cup roasted/unsalted peanuts
7 8-10 dried chilies cut into ½-inch pieces (adjust to taste)
8 1 tablespoon Sichuan peppercorns, lightly toasted and ground
9 1 tablespoon ginger
10 2 teaspoons sesame oil (this is optional though)

STEP BY STEP PROCEDURE

1 In a shallow bowl, combine all the ingredients for the chicken. Cover and let it marinate for 10 minutes, if time allows.

2 Whisk together the sauce ingredients until the sugar dissolves. Set the sauce aside.

3 Heat a large skillet, pan, or wok over high heat. Add 2 tablespoons of cooking oil and allow it to heat up. Then, add the marinated chicken. Stir-fry the chicken for 3-4 minutes, occasionally stirring, until the edges are browned. Remove the chicken from the heat and set it aside.

4 Add the remaining cooking oil to the same pan or wok. Stir in the garlic, ginger, diced chili peppers (capsicums), and Sichuan peppercorns. Stir-fry for 1 minute.

5 Give the prepared sauce a mix, then pour it into the pan/wok. Bring it to a boil while stirring.

6 Once the sauce begins to thicken slightly, add the chicken back into the pan/wok. Mix all the ingredients together, ensuring the chicken is evenly coated and the sauce has thickened (approximately 2 minutes).

7 Stir in the green onions, peanuts, and sesame oil. Toss everything well and continue to cook for an additional 2 minutes to allow the flavors to meld together.

8 Serve the dish immediately with steamed or cooked rice, or enjoy it with fried rice!

9.5 PEKING DUCK

Peking Duck (北京烤鸭) is an iconic dish in Chinese cuisine, and its name pays homage to the city of its origin, Beijing (formerly known as Peking). This culinary masterpiece dates back several centuries. The dish showcases sliced pieces of roast duck featuring irresistibly crispy skin and succulent meat. It is traditionally served alongside thin pancakes, a savory sauce, and julienned vegetables. These components are skillfully assembled into rolls, creating a delightful culinary experience.

INGREDIENTS

1 1 duck - about 2.5kg/5.5lb
2 2 tablespoon fine salt

For the syrup

3 2 tablespoon maltose
4 120 ml hot water - about ½ cup
5 1 teaspoon vinegar

For the stuffing

1 2 stalks scallions
2 1 head garlic
3 2 apples - quartered
4 4 star anise
5 4 bay leaves
6 2 pieces cassia cinnamon

For the sauce

1 3 tablespoon sweet bean sauce (Tian Mian Jiang/甜面酱)

2 1 teaspoon sugar

Other additions

1 Scallions - julienned
2 Peking duck pancakes - homemade or shop-bought
3 Cucumber - peeled and seeds removed, cut into sticks

STEP BY STEP PROCEDURE

1 Gently pat dry the duck using kitchen paper. Rub salt over the skin and inside the cavity. Place the duck on a wire rack with a tray underneath to catch any drips. Let it rest at room temperature at least 1 hour.

2 Bring about 1½ liters (approximately 6 cups) of water to a boil. Carefully pour the hot water over the entire duck, ensuring both sides are covered. You can use a deep tray or do it over a sink. Remove any feather ends from the skin using tweezers.

3 In a bowl, mix maltose with hot water and vinegar until fully dissolved. Brush a layer of this mixture over the duck skin. Refrigerate the duck for 1 hour, then brush another layer of the mixture.

4 Keep the uncovered duck refrigerated on the wire rack, placed over a tray, for 24 to 48 hours.

5 Roasting the Duck:
One hour before roasting, remove the duck from the refrigerator to bring it to room temperature. Stuff the cavity with scallions, garlic, apples, star anise, cassia cinnamon, and bay leaves. Use toothpicks or skewers to seal the cavity openings.

6 Preheat a fan-assisted oven to 200°C/390°F (or 220°C/425°F for a conventional oven). Place the duck on the middle rack of the oven, with the breast side facing up. Position a roasting tray on the bottom rack to collect any dripping fat during roasting. Roast for 15 minutes.

7 Reduce the oven temperature to 180°C/350°F (or 200°C/390°F for a conventional oven). Cover the wingtips and leg ends with aluminum foil. Continue roasting for approximately 60 more minutes.

8 Check the doneness by inserting an instant-read thermometer into the thickest part of the duck, near the breast and inner thigh area. The temperature should be no lower than 74°C/165°F.

9 Serving the Duck: Remove the roasted duck from the oven and let it rest on the counter for 15 minutes.

10 While waiting, prepare the sauce. In a pan, combine ½ tablespoon of the collected duck fat from roasting with sweet bean sauce and sugar. Simmer over low heat until small bubbles appear. Transfer the sauce to a small serving dish and whisk to fully incorporate the sauce and oil.

11 Steam the pancakes for 3 minutes to warm them up if they are cold. Slice the duck into pieces. To serve, spread a little sauce on a pancake, place duck slices, scallions, and cucumber in the middle, and wrap it into a cylinder. Enjoy!

Optional: Cooking Soup
12. After removing most of the meat from the duck, boil the carcass in water to make a soup. You can add Napa cabbage or winter melon to the soup and season with salt and white pepper. This step is optional but adds an extra dimension to the meal.

9.6 ORANGE CHICKEN

Orange chicken is a beloved dish found in many Chinese restaurants. It features bite-sized chicken pieces that are coated in a crispy breading, pan-fried to perfection, and then generously coated in a delectable orange sauce. The sauce is a delightful balance of sweetness, tanginess, and a subtle touch of spiciness. As the name suggests, the star of this dish is the vibrant orange flavor. The distinct citrus taste is achieved by incorporating fresh orange juice and zest into the sauce, creating a delightful burst of citrusy goodness.

INGREDIENTS

Sauce:

1 ¼ cup lemon juice
2 1 ½ cups water
3 ⅓ cup rice vinegar
4 2 ½ tablespoons soy sauce
5 3 tablespoons cornstarch
6 2 tablespoons orange juice

7 2 tablespoons chopped green onion
8 2 tablespoons water
9 1 tablespoon grated orange zest
10 1 cup packed brown sugar
11 ½ teaspoon minced fresh ginger root
12 ½ teaspoon minced garlic
13 ¼ teaspoon red pepper flakes

Chicken:

1 2 large skinless, boneless chicken breasts, cut into 1/2-inch cubes
2 ¼ teaspoon pepper
3 1 cup all-purpose flour
4 3 tablespoons olive oil
5 ¼ teaspoon salt

STEP BY STEP PROCEDURE

1 Gather all the required ingredients.

2 In a saucepan over medium-high heat, combine water, rice vinegar, lemon juice, soy sauce, and orange juice to prepare the sauce. Stir in brown sugar, green onion, orange zest, ginger, garlic, and pepper flakes. Bring the mixture to a boil. Once boiling, remove from heat and let it cool for 10 to 15 minutes.

3 Place the chicken in a resealable plastic bag and pour in 1 cup of the cooled sauce. Seal the bag and refrigerate for at least 2 hours, reserving the remaining sauce.

4 In another resealable plastic bag, mix together flour, salt, and pepper.

5 Remove the chicken (from the marinade) and place it into the bag of seasoned flour. Seal the bag closed and shake thoroughly in order to coat the chicken.

6 Heat olive oil in a large skillet. The heat should be on medium. Cook the coated chicken in the hot skillet until it is browned on both sides.

7 Once cooked, transfer the chicken to a paper towel-lined plate and cover it with aluminum foil. Clean the skillet.

8 Pour the remaining sauce (the one you reserved) into the skillet and then bring to a boil over medium-high heat.

9 In a separate bowl, mix cornstarch and water until it forms a smooth mixture. Stir this mixture into the boiling sauce.

10 Reduce the heat to medium-low, add the chicken back into the skillet, and simmer, stirring occasionally, until the chicken is cooked through, approximately 5 minutes.

11 Serve the orange chicken over rice and enjoy!

CHAPTER 10

FISH

Fish holds a significant position in the culinary traditions of China and various Asian regions, serving as a staple food. Our geographical advantage allows us to boast an abundance of the finest fish species globally, ensuring a plentiful supply for both domestic consumption and the global market.

China encompasses provinces that border seas and lakes, where fish and other forms of seafood dominate as essential food sources. Today, we explore the diverse array of fish recipes originating from these regions.

In these culinary traditions, the most prevalent techniques of food preparation include stir-frying, steaming, and deep frying, which are also commonly employed to cook fish.

10.1. Sweet and Sour Fish
10.2. Pan Fried Honey Teriyaki Salmon Fillet
10.3. Thai Fish Cakes - Tod Mun Pla
10.4. Red Braised Fish Filet (Hong Shao Yu)
10.5. Pan Fried Pomfret
10.6. Pan Seared Fish With Ginger, Scallions, and Soy

10.1 SWEET AND SOUR FISH

In China, Sweet and Sour Fish holds a remarkable reputation as a beloved and widely consumed dish, often served whole. This culinary delight is known for its exquisite presentation, often featuring live fish directly from a tank, which contributes to its higher price point.

INGREDIENTS

1 12 ounces cod fillet (340g, rinsed clean, pat dry and cut into 1-inch cubes)
2 ¾ cup all-purpose flour

3 ¼ teaspoon baking powder
4 ⅔ cup cold seltzer or club soda
5 ⅛ teaspoon turmeric powder
6 ½ teaspoon salt
7 3 cups canola oil (for frying)
8 ⅛ teaspoon white pepper
9 ¼ teaspoon sesame oil
10 1 tablespoon cornstarch

FOR THE SWEET AND SOUR SAUCE:

1 ¼ cup red onion (cut into a 1-inch dice)
2 ⅓ cup water
3 1 tablespoon ketchup
4 2 tablespoons sugar
5 3/4 cup canned pineapple chunks
6 ¾ cup pineapple juice from the can
7 2 ½ tablespoons red wine vinegar
8 ¼ teaspoon salt
9 ¼ cup red bell peppers (cut into a 1-inch dice)
10 1 1/2 tablespoons cornstarch (mixed into a slurry with 2 tablespoons water)
11 ¼ cup green bell peppers (cut into a 1-inch dice)

INGREDIENTS

1 Ensure that your fish fillet is thoroughly cleaned and dried to achieve a delightfully crispy texture when fried. Heat 3 cups of oil in a small pot, conserving oil, until it reaches 380 degrees F. You can use a thermometer or test the temperature by dropping a small amount of batter into the oil. The batter should rise immediately to the surface and turn a light golden brown, rather than browning instantly.

2 Prepare the batter by combining all the dry ingredients: flour, baking powder, cornstarch, salt, turmeric, and white pepper. When you are ready to fry, add sesame oil and cold seltzer water to the dry ingredients and mix until the batter becomes smooth.

3 Dip the fish fillets into the batter, ensuring they are evenly coated while allowing any excess batter to drip off (excessive batter may result in doughy clumps). Carefully place each piece of fish into the oil one at a time, making sure they do not stick together. Fry the fish in batches, avoiding overcrowding, for approximately 3-4 minutes or until golden brown.

4 Use a slotted spoon to remove the fried fish from the oil and transfer them to a cooling rack positioned over a baking sheet to drain excess oil. Repeat this process until all the fish has been fried.

5 In a separate wok or skillet, heat two teaspoons of the frying oil over high heat. Add onions and peppers, stir-frying for 30 seconds, then incorporate the ketchup. Continue frying for an additional 20 seconds to enhance the color and depth of flavor in the sweet and sour sauce.

6 Introduce pineapple, pineapple juice, red wine vinegar, water, salt, and sugar to the wok, stirring to combine. Allow the liquid to come to a low simmer for 2 minutes. While the sweet and sour sauce is still simmering, gradually stir in the cornstarch slurry until the sauce thickens enough to coat the back of a spoon.

7 If the fried fish fillets have softened, you can refry them in batches in oil heated to 400°F for 30 seconds. The higher
temperature compensates for the cooling effect caused by adding a larger batch of fish to the oil.

8 Once the fish is ready, carefully place it into the wok, gently folding it into the sauce with three or four scooping motions until the pieces are lightly coated. Plate the dish and serve immediately!

10.2 PAN FRIED HONEY TERIYAKI SALMON FILLET

Prepare to indulge in the ultimate delight of Pan Fried Honey Teriyaki Salmon Fillet. This dish harmoniously combines a crispy exterior with a tender, juicy interior, resulting in an explosion of flavors that will leave your taste buds in awe. The umami flavors will serenade your palate from the very first bite. The best part? This recipe is quick and hassle-free, making it ideal for a busy weeknight.

INGREDIENTS

1 2 tbsp potato starch or cornstarch
2 1/3 cup soy sauce
3 2 tbsp honey
4 1 tbsp rice wine
5 2 4-oz salmon fillet
6 1 tbsp julienned, sliced, or grated ginger

STEP BY STEP PROCEDURE

1 Begin by preparing the salmon fillet. To maximize the absorption of the delightful teriyaki flavors, score the flesh. Use a knife to create a cross-hatch pattern by making a lengthwise cut and several crosswise cuts. The slices should be deep but avoid cutting through the skin just to keep the fillet together.

2 Proceed to marinate the salmon. Mix together soy sauce, honey, rice wine, and ginger. Transfer the marinade into a resealable plastic bag. Place the scored salmon fillet into the bag, ensuring it is fully immersed in the marinade. Allow it to marinate for 10 minutes, then flip the bag to tenderize the other side of the salmon for an additional 10 minutes.

3 Coat the fillet with potato starch. Sprinkle potato starch evenly on your work surface or use a plate. Remove the salmon from the marinade and lightly press it into the starch, ensuring both sides are thinly and evenly coated. This will create a deliciously crispy exterior.

4 Heat a couple of tablespoons of your preferred cooking oil in a pan over medium heat. Once the oil shimmers, carefully place the salmon into the pan with the skin side down. Cook the fish

uncovered for approximately 5 minutes, then gently flip it and cook for an additional 5 minutes. Finally, transfer the cooked salmon to a plate and serve it hot!

10.3 THAI FISH CAKES- TOD MUN PLA

These red-curry-flavored fish cakes are a beloved and ubiquitous dish in Thailand. The recipe itself is delightfully straightforward, with the main challenge lying in selecting the perfect fish. Opting for a tender variety will yield excellent results, as the texture of the fish cakes corresponds to the firmness of the fish. Personally, I prefer a softer consistency, and basa fish worked wonderfully for me. If the fish available to you is on the firmer side, consider incorporating 1-2 additional egg yolks into the mixture to help tenderize it.

The accompanying dipping sauce bears similarities to the readily available "sweet chili sauce" found on grocery store shelves, and you can certainly use it as a base if you're feeling pressed for time. However, taking the extra step to prepare the sauce from scratch truly elevates the dish and sets it apart.

INGREDIENTS

1 350 g tender fish meat, dried thoroughly if thawed from frozen
2 2-3 tablespoon red curry paste
3 5 kaffir lime leaves, finely julienned
4 1 tsp sugar
5 ½ cup long beans
6 ⅓ cup Thai basil or holy basil, sliced into ribbons if it is large
7 1 egg yolk
8 Fish sauce, as necessary.

DELICIOUS CHILLI DIPPING SAUCE

1 1 big and red chilli pepper. You can also use spur chilli (prik chee fah)
2 Thai chilies. This is optional though.
3 ½ cup of sugar
4 Cucumber slice. This is for serving
5 ⅓ cup of white vinegar, cane vinegar or rice vinegar
6 3 cloves garlic
7 ½ tsp salt
8 3 Tbsp water

Optional additions for the dipping sauce: roasted crushed peanuts, sliced shallots

STEP BY STEP PROCEDURE

1 Let's start with the dipping sauce:
Place the chillies, salt, vinegar, water, garlic and auger in a blender. Blend until smooth, using a low speed if you prefer some chili seeds and pieces for a visually appealing sauce.
Pour the blended mixture into a small pot and bring it to a simmer. Allow it to simmer for about 3-5 minutes, or until it reaches a thin syrup-like consistency.

Bear in mind that as the sauce cools, it thickens. If it becomes too thick after cooling, you can add more water. Set the sauce aside until you're ready to use it.

Tip: If you only need a portion of the dipping sauce for serving, the remaining sauce, without the cucumber, shallots, and peanuts, can be sealed and stored in the fridge for months.

2 Now, let's move on to the fish cakes:In a food processor, combine the fish, curry paste, egg yolk, and sugar. Process them all until they are fine. Ensure to scrape down the sides if necessary. Keep processing for some minutes until the fish becomes firm. It mist be firm enough to hold its shape when spooned. You can then cook a small amount of the mixture to taste for salt and spice. Adjust the flavours by adding more curry paste for a stronger curry taste or spiciness, keeping in mind that it adds saltiness as well. If you want more saltiness, add a little fish sauce.

Then, transfer the fish paste to a mixing bowl and add Kaffir lime leaves, chopped long beans and Thai basil. Stir well until all the ingredients are thoroughly combined.

Prepare your station by having a bowl of cold water and some paper towels next to the stove. Follow these steps based on your preferred cooking method:

3 For deep-frying: Heat a skillet over medium heat and add enough oil to coat the bottom. Moisturise your hands and a tablespoon in the cold water. Then, scoop a tablespoon of fish paste with the wet spoon and gently pat it to form a patty in your hands. Place the patties in the preheated skillet and fry until browned on both sides, approximately 2 minutes per side. You may need to add more oil as you continue frying if necessary.

4 For pan-frying: Heat a skillet over medium heat and add enough oil to coat the bottom. Moisturise your hands and a tablespoon in the cold water. Then, scoop a tablespoon of fish paste with the wet spoon and gently pat it to form a patty in your hands. Place the patties in the preheated skillet and fry until browned on both sides, approximately 2 minutes per side. You may need to add more oil as you continue frying if necessary.

5 To serve, stir shallots, cucumber slices and peanuts into the dipping sauce. Serve the fish cakes with the prepared dipping sauce.

10.5 PAN FRIED POMFRET

If you prioritize your health and prefer non-deep-fried options, Crispy Pan Fried Pomfret is an excellent choice for you. This dish is ideal for post-workout meals due to its high protein content.

In this recipe, pomfret pieces are marinated with a blend of spices and then shallow fried using minimal oil. The result is a crispy texture that satisfies your taste buds without compromising your health goals. Pair it with a refreshing salad, and you have a perfect dinner option for your wholesome evenings. Additionally, it can be served as a delectable side dish alongside your main meal.

INGREDIENTS

1 1 Pomfret fish , cut into 1 inch size pieces
2 1 teaspoon Salt , + Extra for pomfret pieces

3 1/2 Cup Sooji (Semolina/ Rava) , or breadcrumbs
4 2 tablespoons Oil

For the Fish Batter:

1 5 sprig Coriander (Dhania) Leaves , chopped
2 1 Inch Ginger
3 3 Whole Black Peppercorns
4 3 cloves Garlic
5 3 Cloves (Laung)
6 1/2 teaspoon Turmeric powder (Haldi)
7 4 Dry Red Chillies
8 1 teaspoon Fennel seeds (Saunf)
9 Tamarind , Marble size ball

STEP BY STEP PROCEDURE

1 To start preparing the Crispy Pan Fried Pomfret Recipe, begin by washing the Pomfret thoroughly with water. Drain off any excess water and sprinkle some salt over the fish. Set it aside for 5 minutes.

2 In a mixer grinder, combine coriander leaves, fennel seeds, whole black peppercorns, cloves, turmeric powder, dry red chillies, garlic, ginger, and tamarind.

3 Grind all the spices into a smooth batter for the fish, adding approximately 1/3 cup of water. Add a teaspoon of salt to the paste and mix well.

4 Apply this batter or paste to the pomfret pieces, ensuring they are evenly coated. Allow the fish to marinate in the paste for about 10 minutes.

5 Heat a skillet and add oil. Coat the marinated pomfret pieces with semolina on both sides, ensuring they are well coated.

6 Place the coated pomfret pieces in the hot skillet. Fry them over medium heat for approximately 3 to 4 minutes.

7 Flip the pieces to fry the other side. Once they turn golden brown and crispy, switch off the heat and transfer them to a serving plate. Enjoy this flavorful and crispy pomfret masala fry as an appetizer.

8 Serve the Crispy Pan Fried Pomfret alongside Prawns Coconut Curry and Steamed Rice for a satisfying weekday meal.

10.6 PAN SEARED FISH WITH GINGER, SCALLIONS, AND SOY

Fish dishes are known for their simplicity and efficiency in preparation. They are an excellent choice when you're pressed for time but still want a nourishing and flavorful meal.

Typically, the prep work for fish dishes takes around 10-15 minutes, and the cooking time is usually under 5 minutes. This means you can have a delicious fish dish ready to enjoy in just about 15-20 minutes from start to finish. It's impressive how quickly you can create a satisfying and delectable meal with fish.

INGREDIENTS

1 500 gram (1 lb) white flesh fish fillet, cut into bite sizes (Note 1)
2 2 teaspoon cornstarch/tapioca starch
3 4 inch ginger, peeled and thinly sliced
4 3 tablespoon oil
5 1/2 teaspoon sesame oil
6 4 scallion, cut into 2 inch lengths
7 2 teaspoon Shaoxing wine

Sauce

1 1 tablespoon oyster sauce
2 1 tablespoon light soy sauce
3 1 teaspoon cornstarch/tapioca starch
4 2 teaspoon sugar
5 8 tablespoon water/chicken stock
6 1/2 teaspoon ground white pepper

STEP BY STEP PROCEDURE

1 Start by combining the fish fillets with cornstarch and Shaoxing wine. Set aside for a moment.

2 In a separate bowl, prepare the sauce by mixing together chicken stock or water, light soy sauce, oyster sauce, sugar, cornstarch or tapioca starch, and ground white pepper. Set the sauce aside.

3 Heat 2 tablespoons of oil in a wok over medium-high heat. Sauté the ginger and scallions until they become fragrant, which should take around 2 minutes. Remember to reserve some scallions for garnishing later.

4 Add the fish fillets to the wok and sauté them until they are halfway cooked, approximately 30 seconds. Pour in the prepared sauce and continue cooking until the fish is fully cooked, which should take around 1 minute.

5 Turn off the heat and toss in the reserved scallions and sesame oil. Mix everything together well. Transfer the dish to a serving plate and serve immediately.